Rheumatology Drug Review: for Boards and Clinical Practice

© 2026 Donica Liu Baker, MD, FACR

Contents

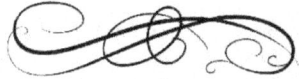

CHAPTER 1 **DMARDs**..9

    Methotrexate (Rheumatrex)..10

    Rasuvo dosing..11

    Leflunomide (Arava)..12

    Sulfasalazine (Azulfidine)..13

    Hydroxychloroquine (Plaquenil)..14

    Chloroquine (Aralen)...15

    Quinacrine (Atabrine)..16

    Dapsone (Aczone)..17

    Thalidomide (Thalomid)..18

    Minocycline (Minocin)...19

CHAPTER 2 **Immunomodulatory agents**..20

    Azathioprine (Imuran)...21

    Mycophenolate mofetil (Cellcept)..22

    Apremilast (Otezla)...23

    Cyclophosphamide (Cytoxan)..24

    Cyclosporine (Gengraf)...25

    Voclosporin (Lupkynis)...26

    IVIG (Immune Globulin)...27

    Plasmapheresis (PLEX)...28

CHAPTER 3	**JAK inhibitors**	29
	Tofacitinib (Xeljanz)	30
	Baricitinib (Olumiant)	31
	Upadacitinib (Rinvoq)	32
	Deucravacitinib (Sotyktu)	33
	Nintedanib (Ofev)	34
CHAPTER 4	**Biologics**	35
	Adalimumab (Humira)	36
	Etanercept (Enbrel)	37
	Infliximab (Remicade)	38
	Golimumab (Simponi)	39
	Certolizumab pegol (Cimzia)	40
	Rituximab (Rituxan)	41
	Belimumab (Benlysta)	42
	Abatacept (Orencia)	43
	Anakinra (Kineret)	44
	Rilonacept (Arcalyst)	45
	Canakinumab (Ilaris)	46
	Mepolizumab (Nucala)	47
	Tocilizumab (Actemra)	48
	Sarilumab (Kevzara)	49
	Ustekinumab (Stelara)	50
	Secukinumab (Cosentyx)	51
	Ixekizumab (Taltz)	52
	Bimekizumab (Bimzelx)	53
	Guselkumab (Tremfya)	54

Risankizumab (Skyrizi)...55

Anifrolumab (Saphnelo)...56

Eculizumab (Soliris)...57

CHAPTER 5   **Biosimilars:** *What the Rheumatologist Should Know*........................58

CHAPTER 6   **Gout medications**..63

Colchicine (Colcrys/Mitigare)...64

Allopurinol (Zyloprim)..65

Febuxostat (Uloric)..66

Probenecid (Benemid)..67

Pegloticase (Krystexxa)...68

Lesinurad (Zurampic)...69

CHAPTER 7   **Glucocorticoids**..70

Prednisone..71

Prednisolone (Medrol)..72

Methylprednisolone (Solu-Medrol)..73

Dexamethasone (Decadron)...74

Triamcinolone acetonide (Kenalog)...75

Hydrocortisone (Solu-Cortef)...76

Acthar Gel (Repository Corticotropin)..77

CHAPTER 8   **NSAIDs**..78

Ibuprofen (Advil)..79

Naproxen (Aleve)..80

Indomethacin (Indocin)..81

	Etodolac (Lodine)...82	
	Diclofenac (Voltaren)..83	
	Nabumetone (Relafen)...84	
	Meloxicam (Mobic)...85	
	Celecoxib (Celebrex)..86	
	Low dose aspirin..87	

CHAPTER 9 **Osteoporosis medications**..88

    Alendronate (Fosamax)...89

    Risedronate (Actonel)...90

    Ibandronate (Boniva)...91

    Zoledronic acid (Reclast)..92

    Denosumab (Prolia)...93

    Raloxifene (Evista)..94

    Calcitonin (Miacalcin)...95

    Teriparatide (Forteo)..96

    Abaloparatide (Tymlos)..97

    Romosozumab (Evenity)...98

CHAPTER 10 **Investigational drugs**..99

    Tanezumab..100

    Filgotinib..101

    Brepocitinib..102

    Olokizumab..103

    Nipocalimab...104

    Ianalumab..105

    Rontalizumab...106

  Sifalimumab……………………………………………………………...…107
  Lenabasum…………………………………………………………................108
  CAR T-Cell Therapy…………………………………………………….......109
References………………………………………………..…………………….....…111
About the Author…………………………………….……………………….......125

CHAPTER 1

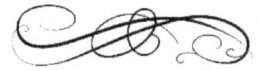

DMARDs

Disease-modifying anti-rheumatic drugs (DMARDs) are medications that change the course of the autoimmune disease for at least one year, with improvements in joint function, decreased synovitis from inflammation, and slowing or prevention of joint damage.

Be sure to tell patients that it might take 3-6 months to achieve a significant response from DMARDs so they do not get discouraged when their pain does not resolve right away.

Abbreviation key:

OA = Osteoarthritis

RA = Rheumatoid arthritis

PsA = Psoriatic arthritis

AS = Ankylosing spondylitis

JIA = Juvenile idiopathic arthritis

SLE = Systemic lupus erythematosus

IBD = Inflammatory bowel disease

UC = Ulcerative colitis

CD = Crohn's disease

Methotrexate (Rheumatrex, Trexall, Rasuvo, Otrexup)

Classification	DMARD
Mechanism of action	Inhibits purine synthesis through inhibition of **dihydrofolate reductase,** which interferes with DNA synthesis, repair, and cellular replication. Also inhibits **AICAR transformylase**, which leads to increases in intracellular AICAR and release of adenosine. **Adenosine** is an inhibitor of neutrophil function and has anti-inflammatory properties.
Major indications	RA, JIA, PsA, AS, reactive arthritis, sarcoidosis.
Other uses	Polymyositis, dermatomyositis, vasculitides, adult-onset Still's disease, SLE, uveitis.
Contraindications	Avoid in renal sufficiency with creatinine clearance < 30 mL/min. Hepatitis B and C infection, cirrhosis, alcoholism. Pregnancy.
Side effects	<ul><li>Oral ulcers (stomatitis), glossitis</li><li>Photosensitivity, alopecia</li><li>Nausea, vomiting, weight loss</li><li>Can worsen migraine headaches</li><li>Hepatic toxicity</li><li>Myelosuppression</li><li>Pneumonitis</li><li>Flu-like symptoms</li><li>Worsening rheumatoid nodules</li><li>Worsening leukocytoclastic vasculitis in seropositive RA patients</li><li>Lymphoma – may be related to EBV</li><li>Teratogenic</li><li>Increased MCV value is typically a sign of compliance with medication</li></ul>
Lab screening monitoring	Baseline: CBC, CMP, hepatitis B and C serologies, CXR. Subsequently: CBC and CMP once a month until reaching a stable dose, then every 3 months.
Dose/route/frequency	Each tablet is 2.5 mg. A typical starting dose is usually 10 mg (4 tablets) once per week, titrated over time to 20 mg once per week and checking labs in between. Take with folic acid 1 mg per day.
Drug interactions	Bactrim
Pregnancy category	X; Women of childbearing age need contraception. MTX should be stopped for 3 months in both males and females before attempting to conceive.
Patient education	Avoid excessive alcohol consumption (recommended amount varies from expert to expert). Avoid live vaccines. Immune response to flu and other vaccines may be blunted.
Other notes	Can test for Methotrexate polyglutamate (MTX-PG) level to determine compliance and ability to achieve therapeutic levels.

Tips on Rasuvo dosing:

Subcutaneous methotrexate can be used when patients are not able to tolerate oral methotrexate due to stomach upset or other side effects. The subcutaneous formulation can also be safely given at a higher dose of 25 to 30 mg once per week and may have better bioavailability compared to the oral methotrexate tablets. Patients should still take folic acid supplementation with subcutaneous methotrexate. Generally, each 0.1 mL of subcutaneous methotrexate equals 2.5 mg (one tablet) of oral methotrexate.

In other words, **each 0.1 cc = 0.1 mL = 10 units = 2.5 mg of methotrexate.**

Here is an easy-to-use conversion table for equivalent doses:

Subcutaneous methotrexate	Oral methotrexate
0.3 mL	7.5 mg
0.4 mL	10 mg
0.5 mL	12.5 mg
0.6 mL	15 mg
0.7 mL	17.5 mg
0.8 mL	20 mg
0.9 mL	22.5 mg
1.0 mL	25 mg

Fortunately, Rasuvo typically comes in prefilled syringes, which is easy for patients to understand and use. The medication has a bright yellow appearance and is administered using an auto-injector.

Leflunomide (Arava)

Classification	DMARD
Mechanism of action	Inhibition of **dihydroorotate dehydrogenase** leads to reduction in de novo synthesis of uridine and decrease in synthesis of pyrimidines. Proliferation of B cells is especially sensitive to reduction of uridine.
Major indications	RA – usually used when Methotrexate is contraindicated or not tolerated.
Other uses	?Lupus nephritis – ongoing research.
Contraindications	Caution in renal insufficiency. Hepatitis B and C infection, cirrhosis. Pregnancy.
Side effects	<ul><li>Nausea, vomiting, diarrhea</li><li>Weight loss</li><li>Hypertension</li><li>Skin rash</li><li>Allergic reaction</li><li>Neutropenia, myelosuppression</li><li>Alopecia</li><li>Hepatic enzyme elevation</li><li>Teratogenic</li></ul>
Lab monitoring	Baseline: CBC, CMP, hepatitis B and C serologies. Subsequently: CBC and CMP once a month until reaching a stable dose, then every 3 months.
Dose/route/frequency	Each tablet is 10 mg. A typical starting dose is 10 mg daily, which can be increased to 20 mg daily if tolerated and labs are normal.
Drug interactions	Rifampin increases the toxicity of Leflunomide. Warfarin is potentiated by Leflunomide.
Pregnancy category	X; Women of childbearing age need reliable contraception.
Patient education	Avoid live vaccines.
Other notes	Leflunomide has a very long half-life. Drug elimination procedure is needed in cases of overdose, toxicity, or desire for pregnancy in males and females. **Cholestyramine** 8 grams TID for 11 days will reduce plasma concentrations of Leflunomide.

Sulfasalazine (Azulfidine)

Classification	DMARD
Mechanism of action	Broken down by colonic bacteria to **sulfapyridine and 5-aminosalicyclic acid.** Beneficial effects are predominantly from the anti-inflammatory properties of 5-ASA, which inhibits leukotriene synthesis and lipoxygenase. Multiple anti-inflammatory and immunomodulatory effects, but exact MOA remains unknown.
Major indications	RA, JIA, PsA, reactive arthritis, AS, IBD-associated arthritis.
Other uses	Ulcerative colitis, Crohn's disease.
Contraindications	**G6PD deficiency**, porphyria.
Side effects	<ul><li>Nausea and vomiting</li><li>Rash, pruritus</li><li>Headache and dizziness</li><li>**Reversible azoospermia** (counsel men on fertility if attempting to conceive)</li><li>Neutropenia</li><li>Hemolytic anemia if patient has G6PD deficiency</li><li>Pulmonary infiltrates with eosinophilia</li><li>Hepatic enzyme elevation</li></ul>
Lab monitoring	CBC, CMP at baseline and monthly for the first 3 months of therapy, then every 3 months afterwards.
Dose/route/frequency	Each tablet is 500 mg. A typical starting dose is 500 mg once or twice daily. Dose can be increased slowly to 1000 mg twice daily and then 1500 mg over time. The maximum daily dose is usually 3000 mg in divided doses. Enteric-coated and delayed-release tablets may be better tolerated with fewer GI side effects.
Drug interactions	Ketorolac
Pregnancy category	D
Patient education	Avoid live vaccines.
Other notes	

Hydroxychloroquine (Plaquenil)

Classification	Antimalarial
Mechanism of action	Increases lysosomal pH and disrupts interaction of peptides with class II MHC molecules and binding of RNA/DNA to **toll-like receptors** (especially TLR7 and TLR9). Decreases production of cytokines and prostaglandins by cells (IL-1, IL-6, IFN).
Major indications	RA, JIA, SLE, discoid lupus, antiphospholipid antibody syndrome, palindromic rheumatism, sarcoidosis, prevention of neonatal lupus.
Other uses	Sjogren syndrome, erosive osteoarthritis, mixed data for CPPD.
Contraindications	Retinopathy. Reduce dose for patients with liver or renal toxicity.
Side effects	<ul><li>Retinal toxicity</li><li>Nausea and vomiting</li><li>Headache, dizziness</li><li>Myopathy, cardiomyopathy, peripheral neuropathy</li><li>Rash, hyperpigmentation of skin</li><li>Prolonged QT interval</li></ul>
Lab and other monitoring	Retinal toxicity monitoring at baseline and then every 12 months.
Dose/route/frequency	Weight based dosing reduces the risk of retinal toxicity. A safe dose is 5 mg per kg of actual body weight per day of HCQ base, usually 200 to 400 mg per day (one 200 mg tablet contains 155 mg of HCQ base).
Drug interactions	Tamoxifen increases risk of retinal toxicity. Cimetidine decreases clearance of antimalarials. Antimalarials increases digoxin levels. Antimalarials decrease the effects of anticonvulsants and amiodarone. Caution with drugs that prolong the QTc interval.
Pregnancy category	C, use if benefits outweigh risks. Considered safe in pregnancy and breastfeeding for SLE patients. Has protective effects against neonatal lupus.
Patient education	May take 4-6 months for patients to feel a response. Obtain baseline retinal eye exam and annual screening. Smoking reduces drug effectiveness by inducing cytochrome P450 enzymes.
Other notes	Also shown to lower lipid levels, decreases degradation of insulin, and prevent thrombosis.

Chloroquine (Aralen)

Classification	Antimalarial
Mechanism of action	Increases lysosomal pH and disrupts interaction of peptides with class II MHC molecules and binding of RNA/DNA to **toll-like receptors** (especially TLR7 and TLR9). Decreases production of cytokines and prostaglandins by cells (IL-1, IL-6, IFN).
Major indications	Cutaneous lupus.
Other uses	Skin rash of dermatomyositis.
Contraindications	Retinopathy. Reduce dose for patients with liver or renal toxicity.
Side effects	<ul><li>Has the **highest risk** for retinal toxicity of all the antimalarials</li><li>Nausea and vomiting</li><li>Headache, dizziness</li><li>Myopathy, cardiomyopathy, peripheral neuropathy</li><li>Rash, gray-black hyperpigmentation of skin</li><li>Prolonged QT interval</li><li>Hypoglycemia</li></ul>
Lab monitoring	Retinal toxicity monitoring at baseline and then every 12 months.
Dose/route/frequency	Use < 3 mg/kg ideal body weight of chloroquine base, around 250 mg/day (500 mg tablets have 300 mg of chloroquine base and 250 mg tablets have 150 mg of base).
Drug interactions	Tamoxifen increases risk of retinal toxicity. Cimetidine decreases clearance of antimalarials. Antimalarials increases digoxin levels. Antimalarials decrease the effects of anticonvulsants and amiodarone. Caution with drugs that prolong the QTc interval.
Pregnancy category	Limited data.
Patient education	Baseline retinal eye exam and annual screening. Smoking reduces drug effectiveness by inducing cytochrome P450 enzymes.
Other notes	

Quinacrine (Atabrine)

Classification	Antimalarial
Mechanism of action	Increases lysosomal pH and disrupts interaction of peptides with class II MHC molecules and binding of RNA/DNA to **toll-like receptors** (especially TLR7 and TLR9). Decreases production of cytokines and prostaglandins by cells (IL-1, IL-6, IFN).
Major indications	Cutaneous lupus.
Other uses	Skin rash of dermatomyositis.
Contraindications	Reduce dose for patients with liver or renal toxicity. **G6PD deficiency.**
Side effects	<ul><li>Notably, **does not cause retinopathy**. Can be combined with chloroquine or hydroxychloroquine without additional retinal toxicity.</li><li>Aplastic anemia – especially if lichen planus rash develops</li><li>Hemolytic anemia in patients with G6PD deficiency</li><li>Nausea and vomiting</li><li>Headache, dizziness</li><li>Myopathy, cardiomyopathy, peripheral neuropathy</li><li>Rash, yellow hyperpigmentation of skin</li></ul>
Lab monitoring	CBC if patient is symptomatic or anemia is suspected. Screen for G6PD deficiency prior to initiation.
Dose/route/frequency	100 to 200 mg/day, made by compound pharmacies.
Drug interactions	
Pregnancy category	Limited data.
Patient education	
Other notes	

Dapsone (Aczone)

Classification	Sulfone
Mechanism of action	Free oxygen radical scavenger that impairs the myeloperoxidase system. Prevents normal mycobacterial utilization of para-aminobenzoic acid (PABA) for the synthesis of folic acid by acting as a competitive antagonist of PABA.
Major indications	Leprosy, dermatoses, skin vasculitis (leukocytoclastic, urticarial, erythema elevatum diutinum, cutaneous polyarteritis nodosa), Behcet's disease, SLE rashes.
Other uses	Relapsing polychondritis, pyoderma gangrenosum, dermatitis herpetiformis.
Contraindications	**G6PD deficiency** (screen all patients before starting, especially those of Mediterranean or African descent).
Side effects	<ul><li>**Severe hemolysis with G6PD deficiency** due to oxidation of glutathione</li><li>Methemoglobinemia</li><li>Leukopenia</li><li>Hypersensitivity syndrome</li><li>Liver toxicity</li><li>Nausea</li><li>Peripheral neuropathy (on high doses)</li><li>TEN</li></ul>
Lab monitoring	CBC and CMP every month for 3 months, then every 3 months subsequently.
Dose/route/frequency	50 to 200 mg PO daily. Taken with 1 mg of folate daily. Topical formulations available.
Drug interactions	Probenecid slows renal excretion of Dapsone.
Pregnancy category	C
Patient education	
Other notes	

Thalidomide (Thalomid)

Classification	DMARD or immunomodulator
Mechanism of action	Has anti-inflammatory, immunomodulatory, and antiangiogenic properties. **Reduces TNF-alpha production by 40%.** Downregulates cell surface adhesion molecules involved in leukocyte migration.
Major indications	Oral and genital ulcerations due to Behcet's disease.
Other uses	SLE skin rashes, erythema nodosum, multiple myeloma.
Contraindications	Pregnancy.
Side effects	<ul><li>Sedation, constipation</li><li>Rash</li><li>**Sensory polyneuropathy** (50%), often progressive and nonreversible</li><li>Venous thromboembolism</li><li>Teratogenicity (phocomelia)</li><li>Notably, not associated with opportunistic infections</li></ul>
Lab and other monitoring	**Baseline EMG/NCS study at baseline** and repeated every 6 months. A decline in sensory nerve action potential by 50% requires discontinuation of the drug.
Dose/route/frequency	50 to 300 mg PO tablet per day.
Drug interactions	Anakinra, clonidine.
Pregnancy category	X; FDA requires strict patient and physician registration for use of this drug because of its known teratogenicity.
Patient education	Notify physician if symptoms of polyneuropathy develop.
Other notes	Lenalidomide (Revlimid) is similar to thalidomide but is potentially less toxic.

Minocycline (Minocin)

Classification	Tetracycline antibiotic
Mechanism of action	Minocycline has demonstrated anti-inflammatory properties such as down-regulation of type 2 nitric oxide synthase (a mediator in collagen degradation), upregulation of interleukin-10 (an inhibitory cytokine in synovial tissue), and suppressive effects on B and T cell function.
Major indications	Antibiotic.
Other uses	Off-label use for rheumatoid arthritis.
Contraindications	Pregnancy.
Side effects	<ul><li>Nausea</li><li>Diarrhea</li><li>Rash, photosensitivity reactions</li><li>Dizziness, lightheadedness</li><li>Headache</li><li>Fingernail discoloration, skin discoloration with long-term use</li><li>Change in taste/dysgeusia</li></ul>
Lab and other monitoring	No specific guidelines.
Dose/route/frequency	100 mg oral tablet twice daily.
Drug interactions	Acetretin, tretinoin.
Pregnancy category	D
Patient education	
Other notes	Infrequent use and lack of new data since 2012.

CHAPTER 2

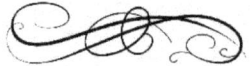

Immunomodulatory Agents

Azathioprine (Imuran, Azasan)

Classification	Immunomodulatory agent
Mechanism of action	Converted to **6-mercaptopurine**, the active metabolite which decreases de novo synthesis of purine nucleotides. This results in cytotoxicity and decreases cellular proliferation. B and T cells are dependent on purine nucleotides for proliferation.
Major indications	RA, SLE, maintenance therapy for Lupus nephritis, polymyositis, dermatomyositis, sarcoidosis.
Other uses	Behcet disease, ANCA vasculitis (maintenance), kidney transplant.
Contraindications	Low or reduced activity of TPMT.
Side effects	<ul><li>Bone marrow suppression</li><li>Nausea, vomiting</li><li>Skin rash</li><li>Increased risk for lymphoma</li><li>Hepatotoxicity</li><li>Isolated hyperbilirubinemia</li><li>Infections – HSV, CMV</li><li>Pancreatitis</li><li>Hypersensitivity syndrome (rash, fever, hepatitis, renal failure within 2 weeks of initiation)</li></ul>
Lab monitoring	Check **TPMT activity or genotype** prior to initiation. Check CBC and CMP at baseline and every 3 months.
Dose/route/frequency	Typical doses range from 50 to 200 mg per day. Start at a low dose, usually 50 mg daily, and increase by 25-50 mg every 1-2 weeks.
Drug interactions	**DO NOT use with Allopurinol or Febuxostat** due to increased risk of toxicity and myelosuppression. Use with sulfasalazine increases risk of leukopenia. Azathioprine may cause warfarin resistance.
Pregnancy category	D; however, when no safer drug is available, use of azathioprine is considered acceptable when patients cannot take alternatives.
Patient education	
Other notes	

Mycophenolate mofetil (Cellcept)

Classification	Immunomodulatory agent
Mechanism of action	Inhibits **inosine-5-monophosphate dehydrogenase** (IMPDH), which decreases synthesis of the purine guanosine. Lymphocytes are dependent on IMPDH, and suppression of this enzyme results in suppression of lymphocyte proliferation and migration. Also has anti-fibrotic activity. Cytokine production is not affected.
Major indications	Lupus nephritis (especially African American and Hispanic patients), cutaneous lupus, scleroderma, myositis, uveitis, vasculitis.
Other uses	Interstitial lung disease in a number of autoimmune diseases such as scleroderma and dermatomyositis, and organ transplant.
Contraindications	Pregnancy.
Side effects	<ul><li>Diarrhea, nausea</li><li>Leukopenia</li><li>Anemia</li><li>Hepatotoxicity</li><li>Infections</li><li>Lymphoproliferative malignancies, especially EBV-associated</li></ul>
Lab monitoring	CBC and CMP every month initially, then every 3 months once on a stable dose.
Dose/route/frequency	A typical dose is 500 to 1500 mg twice daily on an empty stomach. Maximum dose is 100 mg twice daily in patients with renal insufficiency when CrCl is less than 30 mL/min. The 250 mg capsules may be better tolerated than tablets in some patients with GI side effects.
Drug interactions	Cholestyramine and antacids decrease bioavailability of CellCept. Tacrolimus potentiates its effects. Does not interact with warfarin.
Pregnancy category	Avoid in pregnancy due to increased risk of miscarriages and congenital malformations.
Patient education	Female patients need reliable birth control.
Other notes	Myfortic is mycophenolic acid. Some patients may tolerate Myfortic when they have experienced GI side effects with CellCept. Conversion: 360 mg of Myfortic is equivalent to 500 mg of CellCept.

Apremilast (Otezla)

Classification	Immunomodulator
Mechanism of action	Inhibition of **phosphodiesterase 4 (PDE4)** which results in elevation of **intracellular cAMP.** This leads to the reduction of several proinflammatory mediators and cytokines, while increasing the production of anti-inflammatory cytokines such as IL-10.
Major indications	Psoriasis, PsA.
Other uses	Behcet's disease.
Contraindications	Caution in severe renal impairment (CrCl < 30 mL/min).
Side effects	<ul><li>Potential worsening of underlying depression</li><li>Diarrhea</li><li>Nausea</li><li>Headaches</li><li>Upper respiratory infections</li></ul>
Lab monitoring	No specific lab monitoring is required.
Dose/route/frequency	Start at the lowest dose and titrate up slowly. Day 1: 10 mg in AM. Day 2: 10 mg AM and PM. Day 3: 10 mg AM and 20 mg PM. Day 4: 20 mg AM and PM. Day 5: 20 mg AM and 30 mg PM. Day 6 and thereafter: 30 mg PO BID.
Drug interactions	Rifampin, carbamazepine, phenobarbital, phenytoin.
Pregnancy category	Limited data.
Patient education	Report any worsening depression or suicidal ideation.
Other notes	

Cyclophosphamide (Cytoxan)

Classification	Potent immunomodulator
Mechanism of action	Phosphoramide mustard is the major active metabolite, which **alkylates DNA**, resulting in DNA cross-linking and breakage. The result is decreased DNA synthesis and apoptosis, which has the greatest effect on rapidly dividing cells such as lymphocytes.
Major indications	GPA and other vasculitides, lupus nephritis, SLE, ILD in scleroderma.
Other uses	Off-label use in other rheumatic diseases refractory to standard therapy.
Contraindications	Pregnancy, cytopenias.
Side effects	<ul><li>Acrolein, the major metabolic product of this drug, is responsible for increased risk of **hemorrhagic cystitis and bladder cancer.** Give with plenty of fluids.</li><li>Hemorrhagic cystitis occurs more commonly in patients with BK virus.</li><li>Bone marrow suppression.</li><li>Infections, especially herpes viruses.</li><li>**Infertility in women** – premature ovarian failure is dependent on patient age and cumulative dose.</li><li>Azoospermia in men.</li><li>Pulmonary fibrosis or pneumonitis (<1%).</li><li>Reversible alopecia.</li></ul>
Lab monitoring	CBC and UA every month. Nadir in WBC count usually occurs 8-14 days after each dose.
Dose/route/frequency	Oral tablets: 25 mg and 50 mg. IV infusion: 0.5 to 1 gram per m^2 of body surface area. Euro-Lupus dosing: 500 mg IV every 2 weeks for 6 doses. Reduce dose by 30% if CrCl is < 30 mL/min.
Drug interactions	Cimetidine, allopurinol, warfarin.
Pregnancy category	Avoid in pregnancy and lactation.
Patient education	Smoking cessation counseling to reduce risk of bladder cancer. Counsel patients on infertility and family planning.
Other notes	**Mesna**, is a sulfhydryl compound that binds acrolein in the urine and is used for bladder prophylaxis. Using the gonadotropin-releasing hormone analog **Lupron** can be protective against infertility.

Cyclosporine (Gengraf, Neoral)

Classification	Immunomodulator – calcineurin inhibitor
Mechanism of action	Binds to a cytoplasmic protein called **cyclophilin**, which in turn binds to calcineurin. This blocks the interaction of calcineurin with calmodulin, which is necessary to dephosphorylate nuclear factor of activated T cells (**NF-AT**). The end result is decreased transcription of IL-2 and other T cell activation genes.
Major indications	Renal transplant, RA, polymyositis, dermatomyositis, psoriatic arthritis, psoriasis, SLE, lupus nephritis.
Other uses	Uveitis, Behcet's disease, Still's disease, pyoderma gangrenosum.
Contraindications	Renal insufficiency.
Side effects	<ul><li>Nephrotoxicity. Stop cyclosporine if creatinine increases by 30% over baseline, even if it is still in the normal range.</li><li>Hypertension.</li><li>Anemia (pure red cell aplasia).</li><li>Malignancies, usually EBV-related lymphoma.</li><li>Hyperuricemia, gout (switch to tacrolimus which causes less hyperuricemia).</li><li>Bone pain.</li><li>Headaches, tremors, anorexia, hirsutism.</li><li>Hyperpigmentation.</li><li>Rarely hepatotoxicity.</li></ul>
Lab monitoring	Monitor periodic CBC and CMP. Monitor blood pressure and lipid levels.
Dose/route/frequency	25 mg and 100 mg capsules. IV solution 50 mg/mL. Oral solution 100 mg/mL. Initial dosage is usually 2.5 to 4 mg/kg of ideal body weight.
Drug interactions	<ul><li>**Using colchicine and cyclosporine together increases the risk of neuromyopathy.** Patients with severe gout may need to switch from cyclosporine to tacrolimus.</li><li>CYP3A4 inhibitors will increase toxicity of Cyclosporine (erythromycin, clarithromycin, diltiazem, verapamil).</li><li>Taking concurrent NSAIDs, ACE inhibitor, or aminoglycosides will increase risk of renal insufficiency.</li><li>Grapefruit juice increases absorption of cyclosporine and reduces metabolism through inhibition of cytochrome P450.</li></ul>
Pregnancy category	C
Patient education	
Other notes	

Voclosporin (Lupkynis)

Classification	Immunomodulator – novel calcineurin inhibitor
Mechanism of action	Binds to a cytoplasmic protein called **cyclophilin**, which in turn binds to calcineurin. This blocks the interaction of calcineurin with calmodulin, which is necessary to dephosphorylate nuclear factor of activated T cells (**NF-AT**). The end result is decreased transcription of IL-2 and other T cell activation genes.
Major indications	Lupus nephritis – newly approved in 2021.
Other uses	
Contraindications	Renal insufficiency and hypertensive emergency. Not recommended for use in patients with baseline GFR < 45 mL per min. Not recommended for use with severe hepatic impairment.
Side effects	<ul><li>Nephrotoxicity. Reduce dose and reassess within 2 weeks if GFR is reduced from baseline.</li><li>Hypertension.</li><li>Diarrhea.</li><li>Headaches.</li><li>Anemia (pure red cell aplasia).</li><li>Cough.</li><li>Neurotoxicity.</li><li>Hyperkalemia.</li><li>Black box warning for developing malignancies and serious infections.</li></ul>
Lab monitoring	Monitor periodic CBC and CMP. Monitor blood pressure.
Dose/route/frequency	Each oral capsule is 7.9 mg. A typical initial dose is 23.7 mg twice daily. The dose should be adjusted based on GFR and renal function.
Drug interactions	<ul><li>**Using colchicine and voclosporin together increases the risk of neuromyopathy.** Patients with severe gout may need to switch from cyclosporine to tacrolimus.</li><li>CYP3A4 inhibitors will increase toxicity of voclosporin (erythromycin, clarithromycin, diltiazem, verapamil).</li><li>Taking concurrent NSAIDs, ACE inhibitor, or aminoglycosides will increase risk of renal insufficiency.</li><li>Grapefruit juice increases absorption of cyclosporine and reduces metabolism through inhibition of cytochrome P450.</li></ul>
Pregnancy category	Limited data; avoid use in pregnancy.
Patient education	
Other notes	Can be used in combination with mycophenolate mofetil (CellCept).

IVIG (Immune Globulin)

Classification	Immunomodulator
Mechanism of action	The Fc portion of IVIG binds the Fc receptor on reticuloendothelial cells. Has been shown to reduce expression of adhesion molecules on endothelial cells, bind cytokines that cause inflammation, bind and reduce complements, reduce the number of activated T cells, and bind staphylococcal toxin superantigens.
Major indications	Autoimmune thrombocytopenia, Kawasaki disease, dermatomyositis, polymyositis, GBS, CIDP, ITP.
Other uses	Antiphospholipid antibody syndrome (off-label), autoimmune hemolytic anemia and neutropenia (off-label), primary immunodeficiency syndromes.
Contraindications	**IgA deficiency.**
Side effects	<ul><li>In patients with IgA deficiency, there is a risk for anaphylactic reaction.</li><li>Headaches (2 to 20%) – can premedicate with sumatriptan.</li><li>Flushing, diaphoresis.</li><li>Chest tightness.</li><li>Back pain, myalgias.</li><li>Fever, chills, nausea.</li><li>Hypotension.</li><li>Aseptic meningitis.</li><li>Serum sickness.</li><li>Rarely, transmission of infectious agents.</li><li>Renal failure.</li><li>Hypersensitivity reaction.</li><li>TRALI.</li></ul>
Lab monitoring	If patient has baseline renal insufficiency, check renal function 24 hours after infusion.
Dose/route/frequency	1 to 2 grams per kg administered over 1 to 5 days. Usually repeated once per month for a period of 6 months.
Drug interactions	Bacitracin.
Pregnancy category	Limited data.
Patient education	
Other notes	

Plasmapheresis (PLEX)

Classification	Plasma filtration procedure
Mechanism of action	Extracorporeal separation of blood components results in a filtered plasma product. Removes immune complexes and autoantibodies that contribute to the pathogenesis of certain rheumatic diseases.
Major indications	TTP, catastrophic antiphospholipid syndrome, SLE with diffuse alveolar hemorrhage, neuropsychiatric lupus with coma, neuromyelitis optica, GBS, CIDP.
Other uses	ANCA-associated vasculitis with diffuse alveolar hemorrhage or rapidly progressive glomerulonephritis, cryoglobulinemia, Goodpasture syndrome, PANDAS (pediatric autoimmune neuropsychiatric disorders associated with streptococcal infections).
Contraindications	Hemodynamic instability, allergy to fresh frozen plasma or albumin.
Side effects	<ul><li>Infection</li><li>Bleeding</li><li>Patients with hypocalcemia can develop worsening hypocalcemia due to citrate in fluids</li><li>Hypersensitivity to FFP or albumin</li><li>Delayed transfusion reaction</li><li>Hypothermia</li><li>Hypotension due to rapid fluid shifts</li><li>Requires central line placement</li></ul>
Monitoring	Patient's vital signs are monitored every 15 minutes. Signs and symptoms of hypocalcemia are also monitored.
Dose/route/frequency	Removal of 2 to 4 liters of plasma over a 2-hour period. Replacement fluid is usually albumin with saline. Fresh frozen plasma is usually included as part of the replacement solution to reduce risk of infection and bleeding.
Drug interactions	
Pregnancy category	Limited data.
Patient education	Stop ACE inhibitor prior to administration due to increased risk of hypotension.
Other notes	Costs > $5,000 per session

CHAPTER 3

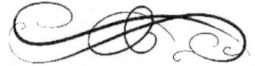

Janus Kinase Inhibitors

Janus kinases (JAKs) are **intracellular proteins** that interact with a number of cytokine and growth factor receptors. Various homodimers and heterodimers can be formed by the four JAKs (JAK1, JAK2, JAK3, and TYK2), with different pairings associated with different cell surface receptors. JAK dimers cause phosphorylation of STAT families, which then translocate to the nucleus. Inhibition of JAKs by the small molecules known as JAK inhibitors cause **decreased phosphorylation of STAT**, which in turn blocks gene transcription of various inflammatory mediators.

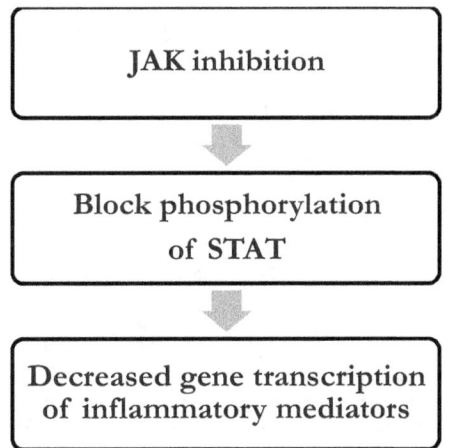

JAK inhibitors in development:
    Filgotinib
    Brepocitinib
    Tyrosine Kinase 2 (TYK2) inhibitors – downregulation of IFN-alpha, IL-12, and IL-23

Tofacitinib (Xeljanz)

Classification	Small molecule; JAK inhibitor
Mechanism of action	Inhibition of JAK intracellular proteins and transduction for a number of cytokine and growth factor receptors. Half-life 3 hours. • Inhibition of JAK1/JAK2 (important for IL-6 and IFN signaling). • Inhibition of JAK1/JAK3 (important for T and B cell signaling). • Inhibition of JAK2/JAK2 (growth factor signaling). • Prevents phosphorylation and activation of STATs (signal transducers and activators of transcription). **Tofacitinib mostly acts on JAK3 preferentially,** and reduces production of IL-2, IL-4, IL-7, IL-9, IL-15, AND IL-21. Acts on JAK1 and JAK2 to a lesser extent.
FDA approvals	RA with inadequate response to MTX, PsA, UC. Psoriatic arthritis, ankylosing spondylitis, juvenile idiopathic arthritis.
Other uses	Ulcerative colitis
Contraindications	History of GI perforation (ask about diverticulitis); see below.
Side effects	• Nasopharyngitis, diarrhea, and headaches • Herpes zoster • Serious and opportunistic infections • Lymphopenia, anemia • Hepatic enzyme elevation • Creatinine elevation • Lipid abnormalities • Malignancy: solid tumors and lymphoma • GI perforations (diverticulitis) • Thromboembolism, particularly with 10 mg BID dosing for patients with ulcerative colitis.
Lab monitoring	CBC and CMP every 3 months. **Lipid panel** every 6-12 months.
Dose/route/frequency	Usually 5 mg tablet PO BID. Extended release is 11 mg QD. Reduce to 5 mg once daily with severe liver or renal disease.
Drug interactions	Avoid azathioprine, tacrolimus, cyclosporine. Tofacitinib dose needs to be reduced by half if patient is taking ketoconazole or fluconazole.
Pregnancy category	Limited data.
Patient education	Shingles vaccine needed prior to initiation. Avoid live vaccines.
Other notes	Blackbox warning for increased cardiovascular events in high risk patients over age 65.

Baricitinib (Olumiant)

Classification	Small molecule; JAK inhibitor
Mechanism of action	Inhibition of JAK intracellular proteins and transduction for a number of cytokine and growth factor receptors. Half-life 12 hours. • Inhibition of JAK1/JAK2 (important for IL-6 and IFN signaling). • Inhibition of JAK1/JAK3 (important for T and B cell signaling). • Inhibition of JAK2/JAK2 (growth factor signaling). • Prevents phosphorylation and activation of STATs (signal transducers and activators of transcription). **Baricitinib acts on JAK1 and JAK2 equally.**
FDA approvals	RA with inadequate response to Methotrexate and TNF inhibitor.
Contraindications	**Renal insufficiency with GFR < 60 mL/min.** Avoid with severe hepatic impairment.
Side effects	• Nausea • Liver enzyme elevation • CK elevation • Thrombocytosis • Herpes zoster infection and other serious infections • Lymphoma and other malignancies • Thromboembolism • GI perforation • Upper respiratory infections • Low blood cell counts
Lab monitoring	CBC and CMP every 3 months. **Lipid panel** every 6-12 months.
Dose/route/frequency	2 mg tablet PO daily.
Drug interactions	Probenecid.
Pregnancy category	Limited data.
Patient education	Shingles vaccine needed prior to initiation. Avoid live vaccines.
Other notes	Blackbox warning for increased cardiovascular events in high risk patients over age 65.

Upadacitinib (Rinvoq)

Classification	Small molecule; JAK inhibitor
Mechanism of action	Inhibition of JAK intracellular proteins and transduction for a number of cytokine and growth factor receptors. Half-life 12 hours. • Inhibition of JAK1/JAK2 (important for IL-6 and IFN signaling). • Inhibition of JAK1/JAK3 (important for T and B cell signaling). • Inhibition of JAK2/JAK2 (growth factor signaling). • Prevents phosphorylation and activation of STATs (signal transducers and activators of transcription). **Upadacitinib acts on JAK1 preferentially.**
FDA approvals	RA with inadequate response to one or more TNF inhibitors. Psoriatic arthritis, ankylosing spondylitis.
Other uses	Atopic dermatitis, ulcerative colitis.
Contraindications	**Renal insufficiency with GFR < 60 mL/min.** Avoid with severe hepatic impairment.
Side effects	• Nausea • Liver enzyme elevation • Thrombocytosis • Herpes zoster infection and other serious infections • Lymphoma and other malignancies • Thromboembolism • GI perforation • Upper respiratory infections • Elevated CK level
Lab monitoring	CBC and CMP every 3 months. **Lipid panel** every 6-12 months.
Dose/route/frequency	15 mg tablet PO daily.
Drug interactions	Probenecid.
Pregnancy category	Limited data.
Patient education	Shingles vaccine needed prior to initiation. Avoid live vaccines.
Other notes	Blackbox warning for increased cardiovascular events in high risk patients over age 65.

Deucravacitinib (Sotyktu)

Classification	Novel tyrosine kinase 2 (**TYK2**) inhibitor
Mechanism of action	Inhibition of intracellular proteins and transduction for a number of cytokine and growth factor receptors. TYK2 differs from other JAK family subtypes in its cytokine signaling specificity. TYK2 primarily regulates **interferon-α, IL-12, and IL-23**. Deucravacitinib achieves a high degree of selectivity by binding to the **regulatory domain** of TYK2, resulting in allosteric inhibition of TYK2 and its downstream functions. Deucravacitinib selectively inhibits TYK2 at physiologically relevant concentrations. At therapeutic doses, deucravacitinib does not inhibit JAK1, JAK2 or JAK3.
FDA approvals	Approved for plaque psoriasis and recently approved in 2026 for psoriatic arthritis.
Other uses	Selective inhibition of TYK2 could potentially provide pharmacological benefits in the treatment of many diseases such as psoriasis, systemic lupus erythematosus (SLE), inflammatory bowel disease (IBD), cancer, and diabetes.
Contraindications	Severe hepatic impairment.
Side effects	<ul><li>Upper respiratory infections</li><li>Herpes zoster and herpes simplex infections</li><li>Mouth ulcers</li><li>Folliculitis</li><li>Elevated CK level; reports of rhabdomyolysis</li><li>Acne</li><li>Hypertriglyceridemia</li><li>Elevated liver enzymes</li><li>Lymphoma</li></ul>
Lab monitoring	CBC and CMP every 3 months. **Lipid panel** every 6-12 months.
Dose/route/frequency	6 mg PO tablet once daily.
Other notes	Mease PJ, Deodhar AA, van der Heijde D, Behrens F, Kivitz AJ, Neal J, Kim J, Singhal S, Nowak M, Banerjee S. Efficacy and safety of selective TYK2 inhibitor, deucravacitinib, in a phase II trial in psoriatic arthritis. Ann Rheum Dis. 2022 Jun;81(6):815-822. Pregnancy data insufficient.

Nintedanib (Ofev)

Classification	Small molecule; tyrosine kinase inhibitor
Mechanism of action	Exerts anti-fibrotic, anti-inflammatory, and vascular remodeling effects through intracellular inhibition of tyrosine kinase. Inhibits platelet-derived growth factor (**PDGFR**), fibroblast growth factor receptor (**FGFR**), and vascular endothelial growth factor (**VEGFR**). Binds competitively to the adenosine triphosphate (ATP) binding pocket of these receptors and blocks the intracellular signaling responsible for the proliferation, migration, and transformation of fibroblasts.
FDA approvals	Systemic sclerosis-associated interstitial lung disease (SSc-ILD). Shown to reduce the decline of FVC.
Other uses	Idiopathic pulmonary fibrosis. Investigations ongoing about ILD in other autoimmune diseases such as rheumatoid arthritis (RA-ILD).
Contraindications	Severe liver disease.
Side effects	<ul><li>Nausea, vomiting, diarrhea, abdominal pain</li><li>Arterial thromboembolic events</li><li>Elevated liver enzymes</li><li>GI perforation</li><li>Increased risk of bleeding</li><li>Skin ulcer</li><li>Cough, Nasopharyngitis, URI</li><li>Fatigue, headaches</li><li>Weight loss, decreased appetite</li><li>Hypertension</li></ul>
Lab monitoring	Monitor liver enzymes periodically.
Dose/route/frequency	150 mg oral capsule every 12 hours.
Drug interactions	CYP3A4 inhibitors (erythromycin), CYP3A4 inducers (carbamazepine, phenytoin, St. John's Wort).
Pregnancy category	Contraindicated in pregnancy due to embryofetal toxicity.
Patient education	
Other notes	Can be used in combination with Mycophenolate mofetil or methotrexate. SENSCIS trial – published in NEJM in May 2019.

CHAPTER 4

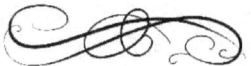

Biologics

Adalimumab (Humira)

Classification	Biologic – TNF inhibitor
Mechanism of action	Human monoclonal antibody that binds both soluble and transmembrane forms of TNF-alpha. Blocks interaction of TNF-alpha with p55 and p75 cell surface TNF receptors. Also lyses surface TNF-expressing cells in vitro and modulates biologic responses responsible for leukocyte migration. Half-life 10-13 days.
FDA approvals	RA, PsA, AS, JIA, Crohn's disease, UC, uveitis.
Other uses	Reactive arthritis, Behcet's disease, relapsing polychondritis, hidradenitis suppurativa.
Contraindications	History of malignancy, demyelinating disease such as multiple sclerosis or GBS, tuberculosis, fungal exposure, class III-IV congestive heart failure.
Side effects	<ul><li>Injection site reactions.</li><li>Opportunistic infections (TB) due to inhibition of granuloma formation, reactivation of latent TB, reactivation of Hepatitis B, atypical mycobacterial and fungal infections.</li><li>Malignancy (particularly lymphomas), melanoma, but no increase in risk of solid tumors.</li><li>Demyelinating syndromes: rare reports of multiple sclerosis, optic neuritis, GBS.</li><li>Development of anti-drug antibodies.</li><li>Worsening of congestive heart failure.</li><li>CK elevation.</li></ul>
Lab monitoring	Some experts recommend periodic lab monitoring with CBC (no guidelines regarding frequency).
Dose/route/frequency	40 mg subcutaneous injection every other week comes as a prefilled syringe or autoinjector pen. Dose can be increased to 40 mg weekly injections if patients report wearing-off effect. Newer citrate-free formulation causes less sting.
Drug interactions	Simultaneous use of methotrexate increases a patient's exposure to adalimumab by 30% and helps prevent the development of anti-adalimumab antibodies.
Pregnancy category	Limited data. Registry reports show slightly increased rate of major birth defects with first trimester use, but no reliable pattern.
Patient education	Possible anaphylactic reaction, rotating injection sites.
Other notes	

Etanercept (Enbrel)

Classification	Biologic – TNF inhibitor
Mechanism of action	Dimeric soluble TNF receptor that binds soluble TNF-alpha and TNF-β. Half-life 3-5 days.
FDA approvals	RA, PsA, AS, JIA.
Other uses	Reactive arthritis, Behcet's disease, relapsing polychondritis, hidradenitis suppurativa.
Contraindications	Uveitis, active infections, inflammatory bowel disease, history of malignancy, demyelinating disease, tuberculosis, fungal exposure, class III-IV congestive heart failure.
Side effects	<ul><li>Injection site reactions.</li><li>Has the potential to worsen inflammatory bowel disease or uveitis. Avoid in these patients.</li><li>Opportunistic infections (TB) due to inhibition of granuloma formation, reactivation of latent TB, reactivation of Hepatitis B, atypical mycobacterial and fungal infections.</li><li>Malignancy (particularly lymphoma), melanoma, but no increase in risk of solid tumors.</li><li>Demyelinating syndromes: rare reports of multiple sclerosis, optic neuritis, GBS.</li><li>Worsening of congestive heart failure.</li><li>**Worsening of uveitis.**</li><li>Drug-induced lupus and autoimmune phenomenon.</li></ul>
Lab monitoring	Some experts recommend periodic lab monitoring with CBC (no guidelines regarding frequency).
Dose/route/frequency	Typical dose is 50 mg subcutaneous injection once a week which comes as prefilled syringes, SureClick autoinjector, or Enbrel Mini cartridges. Can also be used as IM 25 mg twice per week.
Drug interactions	
Pregnancy category	Limited data. Registry reports show slightly increased rate of major birth defects with first trimester use, but no reliable pattern.
Patient education	Possible anaphylactic reaction, rotating injection sites.
Other notes	

Infliximab (Remicade)

Classification	Biologic – TNF inhibitor
Mechanism of action	Chimeric mouse-human monoclonal antibody which binds both soluble and cell-bound TNF-alpha. Half-life 8-9 days.
FDA approvals	RA, PsA, AS, UC, Crohn's disease.
Other uses	IBD-associated arthritis.
Contraindications	History of malignancy, demyelinating disease, tuberculosis, fungal exposure, class III-IV congestive heart failure.
Side effects	<ul><li>Infusion reaction, such as hypotension, headache, nausea, and dyspnea. Can premedicate with Allegra, aspirin, and Solu-Cortef.</li><li>Opportunistic infections (TB) due to inhibition of granuloma formation, reactivation of latent TB, reactivation of Hepatitis B, atypical mycobacterial and fungal infections.</li><li>Malignancy (particularly lymphoma), melanoma, but no increase in risk of solid tumors.</li><li>Demyelinating syndromes: rare reports of multiple sclerosis, optic neuritis, GBS.</li><li>Development of anti-drug antibodies.</li><li>Drug-induced lupus and autoimmune phenomenon.</li><li>Worsening of congestive heart failure.</li></ul>
Lab monitoring	Obtain CBC and CMP before each infusion.
Dose/route/frequency	IV infusions 3-5 mg/kg every 6-8 weeks, which can be increased to as high as 5-10 mg/kg every 4 weeks. Increasing the frequency of infusions is considered more efficacious than increasing the dose.
Drug interactions	Simultaneous use of methotrexate increases a patient's exposure to infliximab by 30%.
Pregnancy category	Limited data in humans. No evidence of toxicity in mice.
Patient education	Possible infusion reactions.
Other notes	Biosimilars:<ul><li>Inflectra (infliximab-dyyb)</li><li>Renflexis (infliximab-abda)</li><li>Ixifi (infliximab-qbtx)</li><li>Avsola (infliximab-axxq)</li></ul>

Golimumab (Simponi or Simponi Aria)

Classification	Biologic – TNF inhibitor
Mechanism of action	Fully human monoclonal antibody that binds soluble and transmembrane forms of TNF-alpha. Median half-life 14 days.
FDA approvals	RA, PsA, AS
Other uses	UC
Contraindications	History of malignancy, demyelinating disease, tuberculosis, fungal exposure, class III-IV congestive heart failure.
Side effects	<ul><li>Injection site reaction.</li><li>Infusion reaction such as hypotension, headache, nausea, and dyspnea.</li><li>Upper respiratory tract infections.</li><li>Opportunistic infections (TB) due to inhibition of granuloma formation, reactivation of latent TB, reactivation of Hepatitis B, atypical mycobacterial and fungal infections.</li><li>Malignancy (particularly lymphoma), melanoma, but no increase in risk of solid tumors.</li><li>Demyelinating syndromes: rare reports of multiple sclerosis, optic neuritis, GBS.</li><li>Development of anti-drug antibodies.</li><li>Worsening of congestive heart failure.</li></ul>
Lab monitoring	Obtain CBC and CMP before each infusion.
Dose/route/frequency	<ul><li>50 mg subcutaneous injection once a month (Simponi).</li><li>IV infusion 2 mg/kg at 0, 4, then every 8 weeks (Simponi Aria).</li></ul>
Drug interactions	Concomitant methotrexate use increases trough concentrations of golimumab by 30%.
Pregnancy category	Limited data.
Patient education	Possible anaphylactic reaction, rotating injection sites.
Other notes	

Certolizumab pegol (Cimzia)

Classification	Biologic – TNF inhibitor
Mechanism of action	Fab fragment of a recombinant, humanized TNF-alpha monoclonal antibody that has been fused to a PEG moiety. Pegylation delays clearance; half-life is 14 days. Cannot cross the placenta due to pegylation and considered safe in pregnancy.
FDA approvals	RA, PsA, Crohn's disease.
Other uses	AS, non-radiographic spondyloarthritis.
Contraindications	History of malignancy, demyelinating disease, tuberculosis, fungal exposure, class III-IV congestive heart failure.
Side effects	<ul><li>Injection site reaction.</li><li>Opportunistic infections (TB) due to inhibition of granuloma formation, reactivation of latent TB, reactivation of Hepatitis B, atypical mycobacterial and fungal infections.</li><li>Malignancy (particularly lymphoma), melanoma, but no increase in risk of solid tumors.</li><li>Demyelinating syndromes: rare reports of multiple sclerosis, optic neuritis, GBS.</li><li>Development of anti-drug antibodies.</li><li>Worsening of congestive heart failure.</li></ul>
Lab monitoring	Periodic CBC (no guidelines regarding frequency).
Dose/route/frequency	400 mg subcutaneous injection at weeks 0, 2, and 4 (loading dose), then 200 mg every 2 weeks (maintenance dose); prefilled syringes.
Drug interactions	Concomitant methotrexate use increases trough concentrations of certolizumab by 30%.
Pregnancy category	Pegylated and considered safe during pregnancy because it cannot cross the placenta.
Patient education	Possible anaphylactic reaction, rotating injection sites.
Other notes	

Rituximab (Rituxan)

Classification	Biologic – B-cell targeted therapy
Mechanism of action	Mouse-human monoclonal antibody against the extracellular domain of CD20 antigen on B cells. All peripheral B cells eliminated within days. Ig levels are preserved. Half-life 19-22 days.
FDA approvals	RA after MTX and anti-TNF failure. ANCA-associated vasculitis (GPA and MPA).
Other uses	SLE, APS, extraglandular Sjogren's syndrome, IgG4 disease, NMO, ITP, autoimmune hemolytic anemia, pemphigus vulgaris, Castleman's disease.
Contraindications	Active infections.
Side effects	<ul><li>Infusion reactions. Use pre-medications.</li><li>Serious and opportunistic infections.</li><li>Viral infections/reactivation: hepatitis B and C, JC virus and PML, herpes zoster</li><li>Hypogammaglobulinemia</li><li>**Late onset neutropenia – occurs an average of 3-4 months post-therapy (cause is unclear)**</li><li>Mucocutaneous reactions (including Stevens Johnson syndrome)</li><li>Hypertension, arrhythmias, MIs during infusions</li><li>No increased risk of CHF, demyelinating disease, mycobacterial infections, or malignancy (except skin cancer)</li></ul>
Lab monitoring	CBC every 2-4 months to **monitor for late onset neutropenia.**
Dose/route/frequency	<ul><li>RA dose: 1000 mg IV infusion repeated once 2 weeks later (500 mg may be just as effective as 1000 mg).</li><li>Vasculitis dose: 375 mg/m^2 IV infusion once weekly for 4 weeks.</li><li>Infusions can be repeated after 6 months.</li><li>Use PCP prophylaxis in patients with vasculitis and lung disease.</li></ul>
Drug interactions	
Pregnancy category	Based on human data, Rituximab can cause adverse developmental outcomes including B-cell lymphocytopenia in infants exposed to rituximab in-utero.
Patient education	
Other notes	

Belimumab (Benlysta)

Classification	Biologic – B-cell targeted therapy
Mechanism of action	Human monoclonal antibody against B lymphocyte stimulator protein (BLyS), also known as **B-cell activating factor (BAFF)**. Decreases peripheral B cell count without affecting Ig levels. Half-life 11-14 days.
FDA approvals	Moderate to severe SLE. Manifestations that respond best are fatigue, rash, and arthritis. Most effective in patients with active serologies (low complement levels, elevated ds-DNA antibodies). Hematologic abnormalities do not respond well. Patients with severe CNS disease were excluded from trials.
Other uses	Lupus nephritis, according to new data.
Contraindications	Active infections.
Side effects	<ul><li>Infections</li><li>Infusion reactions</li><li>Depression and suicide rate mildly increased over placebo</li><li>Nausea</li><li>Hypersensitivity reaction</li><li>Diarrhea</li></ul>
Lab monitoring	No specific guidelines. Some physicians check CBC, CMP with every infusion.
Dose/route/frequency	<ul><li>200 mg subcutaneous injection once per week (not weight based).</li><li>Infusion: Loading dose of 10 mg/kg IV infusion at 0, 2, and 4 weeks. Maintenance dose is 10 mg/kg IV every 4 weeks. No premedications needed.</li></ul>
Drug interactions	
Pregnancy category	Limited data.
Patient education	
Other notes	Initial studies excluded patients with renal and CNS manifestation of SLE. Further studies led to approval of belimumab for lupus nephritis in September 2020. [Furie et al. Two-Year, Randomized Controlled Trial of Belimumab in Lupus Nephritis. NEJM, September 2020].

Abatacept (Orencia)

Classification	Biologic – T-cell targeted therapy
Mechanism of action	Human fusion protein comprising **CTLA4, which binds to CD80/86** on antigen presenting cells, preventing these molecules from binding to their ligand, CD28, on T cells (inhibits co-stimulation and T cell activation). T cells depend on a co-stimulatory signal to become full activated.
FDA approvals	RA, polyarticular JIA with inadequate response to DMARDs.
Other uses	PsA, investigations on ILD and systemic sclerosis.
Contraindications	Active infections.
Side effects	<ul><li>Infusion reactions.</li><li>Infections. Abatacept may be the safest biologic to use in patients at risk for TB. Does not have a black box warning for opportunistic infections.</li><li>Headaches.</li><li>No increased risk of demyelinating disease, CHF, hematologic abnormalities, or autoimmune phenomenon.</li><li>No increased risk of malignancy.</li></ul>
Lab monitoring	No specific guidelines.
Dose/route/frequency	<ul><li>Prefilled syringe: 125 mg subcutaneous injection once per week.</li><li>Infusion dose in adults: based on weight. If < 60 kg, give 500 mg. If between 60-100 kg, give 750 mg. If > 100 kg, give 1000 mg. Loading dose at 0, 2, and 4 weeks, then every 4 weeks.</li><li>Infusion dose in pediatric patients: if < 75 kg, give 10 mg/kg. If > 75 kg, same as adult dosing.</li></ul>
Drug interactions	
Pregnancy category	Limited data.
Patient education	
Other notes	May be the safest biologic to use in patients at risk for TB and other opportunistic infections, as well as patients with a history of cancer.

Anakinra (Kineret)

Classification	Biologic – IL-1 inhibitor
Mechanism of action	Recombinant, non-glycosylated form of the human IL-1 receptor antagonist (IL-1Ra) derived from *E. coli*. Competitively inhibits IL-1 binding to the IL-1 receptor. Half-life 4-6 hours.
FDA approvals	RA, cryopyrin-associated periodic fever syndromes (CAPS), neonatal onset multisystem inflammatory disease (NOMID).
Other uses	Still's disease, Adult onset Still's disease, gout, familial Mediterranean fever.
Contraindications	Active infections.
Side effects	<ul><li>Serious infections</li><li>Neutropenia</li><li>Injection site reactions</li><li>Headache</li></ul>
Lab monitoring	CBC monthly for 3 months, then every 3 months.
Dose/route/frequency	100 mg subcutaneous injection daily.
Drug interactions	Thalidomide, Lenalidomide.
Pregnancy category	B
Patient education	
Other notes	$1500 per month.

Rilonacept (Arcalyst)

Classification	Biologic – IL-1 inhibitor
Mechanism of action	Dimeric fusion protein that incorporates both IL-1 receptor and the receptor accessory protein, targeting both IL-1 alpha and beta. Also known as IL-1 TRAP. Blocks interleukin-1beta (IL-1beta) signaling by acting as a soluble decoy receptor that binds IL-1beta and prevents its interaction with cell surface receptors.
FDA approvals	Familial cold autoinflammatory syndrome (FCAS), Muckle-Wells syndrome (MWS), periodic fever syndromes.
Other uses	Gout, Still's disease, and other cryopyrinopathies (CAPS).
Contraindications	Active infections.
Side effects	<ul><li>Injection site reactions</li><li>Upper respiratory tract infection</li><li>Serious infections</li><li>Lipid abnormalities</li></ul>
Lab monitoring	CBC periodically. Lipid profile at 3 months.
Dose/route/frequency	<ul><li>Pediatric ages 12-17: load with 4.4 mg/kg followed by 2.2 mg/kg subcutaneously once per week.</li><li>Adults: load with 320 mg subcutaneous injection followed by 160 mg subcutaneously once per week.</li></ul>
Drug interactions	Warfarin
Pregnancy category	C
Patient education	
Other notes	$24,000 per month

Canakinumab (Ilaris)

Classification	Biologic – IL-1 inhibitor
Mechanism of action	Human monoclonal antibody targeting IL-1 beta only.
FDA approvals	Familial cold autoinflammatory syndrome (FCAS), Muckle-Wells syndrome (MWS), Still's disease, Adult onset Still's disease, JIA, periodic fever syndromes (HIDS, MKD, TRAPS).
Other uses	Gout and other cryopyrinopathies (CAPS).
Contraindications	Active infections.
Side effects	<ul><li>Nasopharyngitis</li><li>Diarrhea</li><li>Vertigo (10%)</li><li>Headache</li><li>Injection site reactions</li></ul>
Lab monitoring	CBC and LFTs periodically.
Dose/route/frequency	Dosing is weight based:<ul><li>For patient weight 15-40 kg: 2-3 mg/kg subcutaneously every 8 weeks.</li><li>For patient weight > 40 kg: 150 mg subcutaneously every 8 weeks.</li></ul>
Drug interactions	Warfarin
Pregnancy category	Limited data.
Patient education	
Other notes	$8,000 per month.

Mepolizumab (Nucala)

Classification	Biologic – IL-5 inhibitor
Mechanism of action	Humanized monoclonal antibody specific for IL-5; binds IL-5 and stops it from binding to its receptor on the surface of eosinophils.
Major indications	Eosinophilic granulomatosis with polyangiitis (Churg-Strauss).
Other uses	Severe asthma.
Contraindications	Parasitic infections.
Side effects	<ul><li>Headache</li><li>Injection site reactions</li><li>Hypersensitivity reaction</li><li>Herpes zoster</li><li>Patients with parasitic infections were excluded from clinical trials</li></ul>
Lab monitoring	No specific guidelines.
Dose/route/frequency	300 mg subcutaneous injection every 4 weeks for EGPA. 100 mg subcutaneous injection every 4 weeks for severe asthma.
Drug interactions	
Pregnancy category	Limited data.
Patient education	
Other notes	

Tocilizumab (Actemra)

Classification	Biologic – IL-6 inhibitor
Mechanism of action	Human monoclonal antibody that binds to the soluble and membrane-bound forms of the IL-6 receptor. Shown to decrease ESR and CRP levels. Half-life 8-14 days.
FDA approvals	RA, JIA. *Recently approved in 2021 for use in interstitial lung disease associated with scleroderma (SSc-ILD) per phase 3 focuSSed trial.
Other uses	GCA, Takayasu's arteritis, Castleman's disease, relapsing polychondritis, Adult onset Still's disease, SLE. Studied for COVID-19 infection with cytokine storm.
Contraindications	History of diverticulitis, inflammatory bowel disease.
Side effects	<ul><li>Upper respiratory infection.</li><li>Serious and opportunistic infections.</li><li>Herpes zoster.</li><li>Elevated liver enzymes (due to inhibition of anti-apoptotic effects of IL-6 on liver cells).</li><li>Lipid elevations.</li><li>Neutropenia, thrombocytopenia.</li><li>GI perforations.</li><li>Macrophage activation syndrome (seen in 3% of JIA patients on this medication).</li><li>No increase in malignancy, CHF, or demyelinating disease.</li></ul>
Lab monitoring	CBC and CMP monthly until stable dose, then every 6-12 months. Lipid panel every 1-2 months until stable dose, then every 6-12 months.
Dose/route/frequency	<ul><li>Subcutaneous injection: 162 mg injection once per week. If body weight is under 100 kg, decrease to 162 mg every other week.</li><li>Infusion: 4 mg/kg IV once every 4 weeks. Can increase to 8 mg/kg once per month.</li></ul>
Drug interactions	Warfarin, cyclosporine, theophylline, omeprazole, simvastatin.
Pregnancy category	Limited data.
Patient education	Lowers blood levels of OCPs – advise patients about birth control.
Other notes	If Tocilizumab causes liver enzyme elevation:<ul><li>Enzymes between 1-3 times the upper limit of normal: reduce dose.</li><li>Enzymes between 3-5 times the ULN: stop medication until enzymes reduce to <3 times ULN, then restart at a lower dose.</li><li>Enzymes >5 times the ULN: discontinue medication.</li></ul>

Sarilumab (Kevzara)

Classification	Biologic – IL-6 inhibitor
Mechanism of action	Human monoclonal antibody that binds to both soluble and membrane-bound IL-6 receptors and has been shown to inhibit IL-6-mediated signaling through these receptors. Half-life 10 days.
FDA approvals	RA with DMARD failure.
Other uses	Investigations ongoing about GCA. Studied for COVID-19 infection with cytokine storm.
Contraindications	Active infection.
Side effects	<ul><li>Infections</li><li>Low WBC or platelet counts</li><li>Liver enzyme elevation</li><li>Injection site reaction</li><li>Hypertriglyceridemia</li></ul>
Lab monitoring	CBC and CMP periodically.
Dose/route/frequency	150 mg to 200 mg subcutaneous injection every 2 weeks (prefilled syringe or pen).
Drug interactions	
Pregnancy category	Limited data.
Patient education	
Other notes	

Ustekinumab (Stelara)

Classification	Biologic – IL-12 and IL-23 inhibitor
Mechanism of action	Human monoclonal antibody that binds to the p40 subunit of IL-12 and IL-23, preventing their binding to the cell surface receptor chain, IL-12 beta. Downstream effects include inhibition of Th17 response, reduction in TNF alpha, IFN gamma, IL-2, and production of cytokines. Half-life 15-45 days.
FDA approvals	Psoriasis and PsA.
Other uses	UC and Crohn disease.
Contraindications	Active infections.
Side effects	<ul><li>Nasopharyngitis</li><li>Upper respiratory tract infection</li><li>Non-melanoma skin cancers</li><li>Serious infections, especially salmonella, mycobacterial, and fungal</li><li>Injection site reaction, hypersensitivity</li></ul>
Lab monitoring	No specific guidelines.
Dose/route/frequency	<ul><li>Patient weight < 100 kg: 45 mg SC injection initially, followed by 45 mg in 4 weeks, then 45 mg every 12 weeks.</li><li>Weight > 100 kg: 90 mg SC injection initially, followed by 90 mg in 4 weeks, then 90 mg every 12 weeks.</li></ul>
Drug interactions	
Pregnancy category	Limited data.
Patient education	
Other notes	Costs $28,000 to $56,000 per year

Secukinumab (Cosentyx)

Classification	Biologic – IL-17 inhibitor
Mechanism of action	Human monoclonal antibody against IL-17A.
FDA approvals	Psoriatic arthritis, ankylosing spondylitis.
Other uses	Psoriasis.
Contraindications	Active infections.
Side effects	<ul><li>Nasopharyngitis</li><li>Upper respiratory tract infection</li><li>Non-melanoma skin cancers</li><li>Serious infections, especially salmonella, mycobacterial, and fungal</li><li>Injection site reaction, hypersensitivity</li><li>May exacerbate Crohn disease</li></ul>
Lab monitoring	No specific guidelines.
Dose/route/frequency	300 mg subcutaneous injection at weeks 0, 1, 2, 3, and 4 (loading dose). Beginning at week 8, give 300 mg SC once per month (maintenance). For some patients, a dose of 150 mg once per month may be sufficient. IV infusion now available in 2024.
Drug interactions	
Pregnancy category	B
Patient education	
Other notes	

Ixekizumab (Taltz)

Classification	Biologic – IL-17 inhibitor
Mechanism of action	Humanized monoclonal IgG4 antibody that targets interleukin-17A.
FDA approvals	Psoriatic arthritis, ankylosing spondylitis.
Other uses	Psoriasis.
Contraindications	Active infection.
Side effects	<ul><li>Nasopharyngitis</li><li>Upper respiratory tract infection</li><li>Serious infections, especially salmonella, mycobacterial, and fungal</li><li>Injection site reaction, hypersensitivity</li></ul>
Lab monitoring	No specific guidelines.
Dose/route/frequency	160 mg subcutaneous injection once as loading dose, then 80 mg subcutaneously every month thereafter as maintenance dose.
Drug interactions	CYP450 substrates.
Pregnancy category	Limited data.
Patient education	
Other notes	

Bimekizumab (Bimzelx)

Classification	Biologic – IL-17 inhibitor
Mechanism of action	Humanized monoclonal IgG1 antibody that selectively inhibits both interleukin-17A (IL-17A) and IL-17F. Among IL-17 family members, IL-17F is closest in sequence to IL-17A, sharing ~50% structural homology.
Major indications	Psoriatic arthritis, plaque psoriasis, ankylosing spondylitis.
Other uses	Hidradenitis suppurativa.
Contraindications	Inflammatory bowel diseases.
Side effects	<ul><li>Headache</li><li>Opportunistic infections</li><li>Injection site reactions</li><li>Diarrhea, nausea</li><li>Worsening depression or suicidal ideation (four completed suicides were reported)</li><li>Exacerbation of underlying inflammatory bowel disease</li><li>Elevation of liver enzymes</li></ul>
Lab monitoring	Monitor liver enzymes - no specific guidelines on frequency.
Dose/route/frequency	For psoriatic arthritis and AS, the dosing is 160 mg subcutaneous injection every 4 weeks. There is a loading dose for plaque psoriasis.
Drug interactions	Do not combine with other biologics.
Pregnancy category	Insufficient data.
Patient education	Report any depression or suicidal ideation. Monitor mental health.
Other notes	McInnes IB, Asahina A, Coates LC, Landewé R, Merola JF, Ritchlin CT, Tanaka Y, Gossec L, Gottlieb AB, Warren RB, Ink B, Assudani D, Bajracharya R, Shende V, Coarse J, Mease PJ. Bimekizumab in patients with psoriatic arthritis, naive to biologic treatment: a randomised, double-blind, placebo-controlled, phase 3 trial (BE OPTIMAL). Lancet. 2023 Jan 7;401(10370):25-37.

Guselkumab (Tremfya)

Classification	Biologic – IL-23 inhibitor
Mechanism of action	Human monoclonal antibody that targets interleukin-23. Binds selectively to p19 subunit of IL-23, thereby decreasing cytokine and chemokine release. Half-life 15-18 days.
FDA approvals	Psoriatic arthritis, plaque psoriasis.
Other uses	Ulcerative colitis, Crohns disease.
Contraindications	Active infection.
Side effects	<ul><li>Nasopharyngitis</li><li>Upper respiratory tract infection</li><li>Headaches</li><li>Serious infections, especially salmonella, mycobacterial, and fungal</li><li>Herpes simplex infections</li><li>Injection site reaction, hypersensitivity</li><li>Diarrhea, gastroenteritis</li><li>Elevated liver enzymes</li></ul>
Lab monitoring	No specific guidelines.
Dose/route/frequency	100 mg subcutaneous injection at weeks 0 and 4 (loading dose), then every 8 weeks thereafter (maintenance dose). Comes as a prefilled syringe or a One-Press injector.
Drug interactions	CYP450 substrates.
Pregnancy category	Limited data.
Patient education	Avoid live vaccines.
Other notes	Each injection costs about $10,000. Can be administered together with a conventional DMARD such as methotrexate.

Risankizumab (Skyrizi)

Classification	Biologic – IL-23 inhibitor
Mechanism of action	Human monoclonal antibody that targets interleukin-23. Binds selectively to p19 subunit of IL-23 and inhibits its interaction with IL-23 receptor, thereby decreasing cytokine and chemokine release. Half-life is about 28 days.
FDA approvals	Psoriatic arthritis and plaque psoriasis.
Other uses	Ulcerative colitis, Crohns disease.
Contraindications	Active infection.
Side effects	<ul><li>Nasopharyngitis</li><li>Upper respiratory tract infection</li><li>Headaches</li><li>Serious infections</li><li>Fatigue</li><li>Injection site reaction, hypersensitivity</li><li>Eczema (in post-marketing reports)</li></ul>
Lab monitoring	No specific guidelines.
Dose/route/frequency	150 mg subcutaneous injection at week 0 and 4 (loading dose), and then every 12 weeks thereafter (maintenance dose).
Drug interactions	No major drug interactions were identified.
Pregnancy category	Limited data. Increased fetal/infant loss was noted in pregnant monkeys. Clinical significance in humans is unknown.
Patient education	Avoid live vaccines.
Other notes	Can be administered together with a conventional DMARD such as methotrexate.

Anifrolumab (Saphnelo)

Classification	Biologic – novel interferon inhibitor
Mechanism of action	Fully human IgG monoclonal antibody that binds to the subunit 1 of the **type I interferon receptor** and inhibits interferon signaling. Cell signaling by all type I IFNs, including IFNα, IFNβ, IFNε, IFNϰ, and IFNω, is mediated by the type I IFN-α/β/ω receptor (IFNAR). Also induces **internalization of type 1 interferon receptor**, which reduces levels of cell surface available for receptor assembly. Blockade of interferon signaling inhibits downstream inflammatory and immunological processes, including plasma cell differentiation.
FDA approvals	Moderate to severe SLE. Patients with lupus nephritis and CNS lupus were excluded from trials.
Other uses	Possibly scleroderma.
Contraindications	Active infection.
Side effects	<ul><li>Infusion reactions.</li><li>Hypersensitivity reactions.</li><li>Higher rate of herpes zoster infection.</li><li>Upper respiratory tract infections; bronchitis.</li><li>Increased risk for serious and sometimes fatal infections (one death from pneumonia in clinical trials).</li><li>Immunosuppressants may increase risk of malignancies; unknown how much anifrolumab increases such risk.</li></ul>
Lab monitoring	
Dose/route/frequency	IV 300 mg infusion every 4 weeks. Currently only available as an infusion. Subcutaneous formulation is still under development. Dosing is not significantly impacted by renal or hepatic function.
Drug interactions	
Pregnancy category	Limited data.
Patient education	Avoid live vaccines.
Other notes	Can be used in combination with other DMARDs. Patients with active lupus nephritis and CNS SLE were excluded from trials (TULIP-2).

Eculizumab (Soliris)

Classification	Biologic – terminal complement inhibitor
Mechanism of action	Monoclonal antibody that binds C5 and inhibits its cleavage to C5a and C5b, which prevents the generation of the terminal complement complex.
FDA approvals	Hemolytic uremic syndrome with complement-mediated thrombotic microangiopathy, neuromyelitis optica spectrum disorder (NMOSD).
Other uses	Paroxysmal nocturnal hemoglobinuria, myasthenia gravis.
Contraindications	Active infection.
Side effects	<ul><li>Meningococcemia due to inhibition of terminal complements. Requires meningococcal vaccine to be given prior to initiation.</li><li>Headache</li><li>Nasopharyngitis</li><li>Back pain</li><li>Nausea</li><li>Cough</li><li>Fatigue</li><li>Hypertension</li></ul>
Lab monitoring	
Dose/route/frequency	Doses 1-4: 900 mg IV every week for the first 4 weeks. Dose 5: 1200 mg IV one week later. Maintenance dose: 1200 mg IV every 2 weeks thereafter.
Drug interactions	
Pregnancy category	Limited data.
Patient education	Patients should receive meningococcal vaccine at least 2 weeks prior to receiving first dose.
Other notes	$450,000 to $600,000 per year

CHAPTER 5

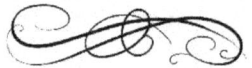

Biosimilars:
What the Rheumatologist Should Know

What is a biosimilar product?

The FDA defines a biosimilar as a biological product that is "highly similar" to the reference product, notwithstanding minor differences in clinically inactive components and with respect to which "there are no clinically meaningful differences between the biological product and reference product in terms of the safety, purity, and potency of the product." The World Health Organization defines a biosimilar as a "biological product that is similar in terms of quality, safety, and efficacy to an already licensed reference biotherapeutic product."

To qualify as a biosimilar, one requirement is that the primary amino acid sequence must be identical to the originator biologic. There may be differences in higher order protein and biochemical structure between the biosimilar and originator biologic. These differences are extensively analyzed to determine that they are not expected to be clinically relevant. Biosimilars have the same dosing schedule and route of administration as the originator biologic.

Is 'biosimilar" the same as "generic"?

No, the term "generic medication" is used to describe small molecules which are chemicals with a fixed and identical molecular formula, such as antihistamines, aspirin, statins, etc. These can be produced at very low prices without enduring extensive clinical trials. On the other hand, "biosimilars" have a complex protein structure and is a biological product from a living organism that must undergo clinical trials to prove their similarity to the reference product.

What are factors to consider when evaluating similarity?
- Manufacturing process
- Physicochemical properties
- Functional activities
- Receptor binding
- Immunochemical properties
- Impurities
- Reference product and standards
- Final drug product
- Stability
- Immunogenicity

What is the process of biosimilar development?
1. Characterization
    a. Physicochemical characteristics
    b. Post-translational modifications – for example, glycosylation

c. Pharmacokinetics
   d. Effector functions

2. Pre-clinical studies

   a. Biosimilar manufacturers try to match the originator's critical quality attributes as closely as possible.

3. Clinical studies
   a. Phase I: 15 to 30 health human volunteers are subjected to the drug at different dosages to determine its risk profile.
   b. Phase II: involves up to 200 patients at optimized dose.
   Expensive Phase II trials may be skipped in development of biosimilars which is an abbreviated pathway compared to originator development. Dose ranging is not necessary. This may save money for the pharmaceutical company leading to cost savings for the healthcare system.
   c. Phase III: enrolls up to 3,000 patients to confirm safety and efficacy in a sensitive patient population.

What does the term "interchangeability" refer to?

This term refers to "the possibility of exchanging one medicine for another medicine that is expected to have the same clinical effect." Interchangeability is defined by statute in the USA to mean that the "biological product may be substituted for the reference product without the intervention of the healthcare provider who prescribed the reference product," and this would enable pharmacy-medicated substitution where state laws allow. This requires an additional standard beyond biosimilarity defined in the statute and the FDA is drafting guidance on "Considerations in Demonstration Interchangeability with a Reference Product."

The FDA defines an interchangeable biosimilar as one that "can be expected to produce the same clinical result as the reference product in any given patient, and if the biologic is administered more than once to an individual, the risk in terms of safety or diminished efficacy of alternating or switching between the use of the biologic and the reference product is no greater than the risk of using the reference product without such alternation or switch."

What are the expected cost savings for using branded biosimilars?

There is a common misconception that biosimilars are "generic" versions of biologic drugs and much cheaper. The reality is that biosimilars are still branded by pharmaceutical companies – they cost less than the original biologic but can still be quite costly. Biosimilars could provide savings and efficiencies for healthcare systems, but these savings are not expected to as dramatic as for generic drugs, since it still takes a pharmaceutical company about 8-10 years to develop a biosimilar and a cost of $100-200 million dollars on average.

In the USA, it has been projected that biosimilars will lead to $44.2 billion reduction in biologic spending over a 10-year period, based on an estimated 35% price reduction. Savings for the healthcare system could lead to expansion of patient access to biologic treatments. For example, a budget analysis of the rituximab biosimilar in European countries estimated a savings of 56.82 million Euros over a one-year period, which would expand patient access to rituximab treatment for an additional 2263 patients with non-Hodgkins lymphoma.

Biosimilars are required to be priced at a discount relative to their reference products, currently at about 30% in Europe. This discount is likely to increase to 50% or more in the US eventually. For example, compared to Remicade which costs about $940 per vial, its corresponding biosimilar Inflectra costs about $525 per vial which is a 44% discount. Introduction of biosimilars can also promote price competition within the market over time.

The amount of money each individual patient saves out-of-pocket varies will depend on type of insurance (commercial versus Medicare/Medicaid) and use of the copay cards for commercial insurance, as well as route of administration (subcutaneous injection versus infusion). For example, a commercially insured patient who receives Humira for $0 or $5 per month with the copay card has very little incentive to switch to a biosimilar. On the other hand, a Medicare patient who is receiving a biologic infusion may see greater cost savings by switching to a biosimilar, and insurance companies will definitely save money in both scenarios. Patient assistance programs are still available for patients who aren't able to afford these drugs.

What do the random letters mean at the end of a biosimilar name?

In 2017, the FDA introduced a regulatory framework where the nonproprietary name of a biosimilar should consist of a "core name" followed by a four-letter suffix. This proposal calls for incorporation of a "biologic qualifier" that comprises of four random consonants. Thus, all biosimilars have a core name followed by a dash and four random letters to distinguish between different biosimilars. For example, "infliximab-qbtx," "adalimumab-adaz," or "etanercept-ykro" are names assigned to different biosimilars.

What are "biobetters"?

A biobetter has improved characteristics of the innovator or originator molecule. For example, one could argue that Humira was a "biobetter" for Remicade because it is a TNF inhibitor that reduced immunogenicity by humanizing the antibody. The most common modification is the addition of the polytheylene glycol (PEG) to the Fc region of the mAb which prolongs renal clearance and gives more time for the mAb to stay in the blood – for example the production of certolizumab pegol (Cimzia).

How do I talk to my patients about biosimilars?

Patients may have a number of questions and concerns about receiving or switching to biosimilar treatments. They may wonder how safe the biosimilar is and whether it will be as effective or not. Patients may perceive that because a drug is less expensive, it is less effective, or inferior compared to a more expensive drug. They may experience a "nocebo effect" which is when a negative expectation of a treatment leads to potentially worse outcomes.

Healthcare providers should have open and honest discussions with patients about biosimilars and avoid using overly technical language and medical jargon. Here are some key summary points to share with your patients regarding biosimilars:
- Biosimilars are highly similar to the originator biologic in terms of safety, purity, and efficacy.
- The primary structure is required to be identical to the originator biologic, but minor structural and biochemical characteristics may be different. These differences are not considered to impact clinical efficacy and safety.
- Biosimilars are not generic versions of biologic drugs.
- Biosimilars are regulated by the FDA and studied in clinical trials to ensure that they are as safe and effective as the original biologic when used in practice.

Further resources and printable handouts on biosimilars to give to your patients:
- US FDA: https://www.fda.gov/drugs/biosimilars/biosimilar-basics-patients
- European Commission: https://ec.europa.eu/docsroom/documents/26643
- National Rheumatoid Arthritis Society: https://nras.org.uk/resource/biosimilars

CHAPTER 6

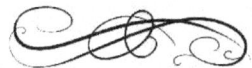

Gout Medications

Medications that help <u>lower</u> serum uric acid levels:

- Amlodipine
- Losartan
- High dose aspirin

Medications that <u>raise</u> uric acid levels:

- Hydrochlorothiazide
- Furosemide
- Low dose aspirin

Colchicine (Colcrys, Mitigare)

Classification	Alkaloid derivative from *Colchicum autumnale* plant
Mechanism of action	Binds to and disrupts tubulin dimers on neutrophils, preventing cytoskeleton assembly into microtubules. Prevents activation, degranulation, and migration of neutrophils. Also inhibits phospholipase A2, which inhibits formation of prostaglandins and leukotrienes. Has no effect on serum urate levels or urate metabolism. Half-life 4 hours.
Major indications	Gout – acute attacks and prophylaxis. Works the best within first 24-48 hours of acute gout flare.
Other uses	Pseudogout, Familial Mediterranean fever, complex aphthosis, acute sarcoid arthritis.
Contraindications	Caution with renal insufficiency and severe liver disease.
Side effects	<ul><li>GI: nausea, vomiting, diarrhea, rarely hemorrhagic gastroenteritis.</li><li>Bone marrow suppression – possible thrombocytopenia, leukopenia.</li><li>**Neuromyopathy**, with elevated CK, proximal muscle weakness, peripheral neuropathy. Muscle biopsy is characteristic with lysosomal vacuoles.</li><li>Alopecia.</li><li>Oligospermia, amenorrhea.</li><li>CNS dysfunction.</li><li>Transient lactose intolerance.</li></ul>
Lab monitoring	Periodic CBC and BMP to assess for cytopenias and renal function.
Dose/route/frequency	0.6 mg tablets or capsules once daily or twice daily with normal renal function. Dose is lowered depending on renal function.
Drug interactions	Interacts with **CYP 3A4** inhibitors: clarithromycin, erythromycin, ketoconazole, ritonavir, calcium channel blockers. Combining colchicine with statins increases risk of myopathy. **Avoid with cyclosporine (increases risk of neuromyopathy).** Tacrolimus is less dangerous.
Pregnancy category	C? Published animal reproduction and development studies indicate that colchicine causes embryofetal toxicity and altered postnatal development at exposures within or above the clinical therapeutic range.
Patient education	Avoiding lactose may help with diarrhea.
Other notes	

Allopurinol (Zyloprim)

Classification	Anti-hyperuricemic agent – xanthine oxidase inhibitor
Mechanism of action	Blocks uric acid synthesis by acting as a hypoxanthine analog and inhibiting **xanthine oxidase**, the final enzyme involved in the production of uric acid. Inhibits conversion of hypoxanthine to xanthine to uric acid. Oxipurinol is the active metabolite which can be measured to assess compliance.
Major indications	Recurrent gout with urate overproduction, nephrolithiasis, renal insufficiency, or tophi.
Other uses	Prophylaxis against tumor lysis syndrome, Lesch-Nyhan syndrome, hyperuricemia secondary to myeloproliferative disorders.
Contraindications	Do not start during an acute attack of gout. Renally excreted - caution with severe renal insufficiency.
Side effects	<ul><li>Can cause an acute gouty attack</li><li>Rash, especially if taken with ampicillin or amoxicillin</li><li>Nausea, diarrhea, headache</li><li>Abnormal liver enzymes</li><li>**Allopurinol hypersensitivity syndrome** – rash, fever, eosinophilia, hepatic necrosis, leukocytosis, and renal failure. Treatment is with high dose steroids and hemodialysis to remove oxipurinol, the active metabolite.</li><li>Bone marrow suppression</li><li>Peripheral neuropathy</li><li>TEN, Stevens Johnson syndrome</li><li>Interstitial nephritis</li><li>Cataracts</li><li>Oxipurinol xanthine nephrolithiasis</li></ul>
Lab monitoring	Check renal function prior to starting. For patients of Korean, Chinese, or Thai descent – check **HLA-B*5801** prior to starting due to risk of allopurinol hypersensitivity syndrome.
Dose/route/frequency	Start at 100 mg daily and increase by 100 mg every month as tolerated to 300 mg daily. Dosage should be lowered with renal insufficiency and increased very gradually.
Drug interactions	**Avoid with azathioprine and 6-mercaptopurine** (both are also metabolized by xanthine oxidase) due to increased risk of bone marrow suppression and neutropenia. Also interacts with ampicillin, amoxicillin, thiazide diuretics, cyclophosphamide, warfarin, cyclosporine.
Pregnancy category	Limited data because women of reproductive age don't usually require treatment with allopurinol.
Patient education	
Other notes	Can be given with Probenecid.

Febuxostat (Uloric)

Classification	Anti-hyperuricemic agent – xanthine oxidase inhibitor
Mechanism of action	Blocks uric acid synthesis by selectively inhibiting **xanthine oxidase**, the final enzyme involved in the production of uric acid. Inhibits conversion of hypoxanthine to xanthine to uric acid.
Major indications	Recurrent gout with urate overproduction, nephrolithiasis, renal insufficiency, or tophi.
Other uses	Prophylaxis against tumor lysis syndrome, Lesch-Nyhan syndrome, hyperuricemia secondary to myeloproliferative disorders.
Contraindications	Do not start during an acute attack of gout. Metabolized by the liver - avoid with severe liver disease. Avoid with severe renal insufficiency, CrCl < 30 mL/min.
Side effects	• Can cause an acute gouty attack. • Black box warning for increased cardiovascular risk and higher rate of death due to cardiovascular events (sudden cardiac death) compared to allopurinol.
Lab monitoring	Check CMP periodically.
Dose/route/frequency	Start at 40 mg per day and increase gradually to 80 to 120 mg per day. No need to decrease dose if GFR is > 30 mL/min.
Drug interactions	**Avoid with azathioprine and 6-mercaptopurine** (both are also metabolized by xanthine oxidase) due to increased risk of bone marrow suppression and neutropenia. Also interacts with theophylline.
Pregnancy category	Limited data.
Patient education	
Other notes	Much more expensive than Allopurinol. Should only be used in patients who have failed Allopurinol or cannot tolerate it.

Probenecid (Benemid)

Classification	Anti-hyperuricemic agent – uricosuric
Mechanism of action	Increases renal excretion of uric acid by inhibiting **URAT1** and **GLUT9** transporters in the proximal tubule of the kidneys. Depends on adequate renal function in order to work well. Half-life 6-12 hours.
Major indications	Chronic gout.
Other uses	
Contraindications	Never start during an acute gout attack. Avoid with severe renal insufficiency CrCl < 30 mL/min.
Side effects	<ul><li>Can cause an acute gouty attack.</li><li>Urate nephropathy.</li><li>Urate nephrolithiasis.</li><li>Nausea, low appetite.</li><li>Dermatitis.</li><li>Headache, flushing.</li><li>Rarely anaphylaxis, cytopenias, or nephrotic syndrome.</li></ul>
Lab monitoring	Periodic BMP to assess renal function.
Dose/route/frequency	Start with 250 mg tablets twice daily. Increase to 500 mg twice daily after one week. Gradually increase as needed to 3000 mg per day in divided doses.
Drug interactions	Penicillin, dapsone, methotrexate, indomethacin, heparin.
Pregnancy category	B
Patient education	
Other notes	There is a combination formulation with both Probenecid and Colchicine together in one tablet.

Pegloticase (Krystexxa)

Classification	Anti-hyperuricemic agent
Mechanism of action	Recombinant, pegylated, uricase enzyme. Humans possess the gene for the uricase enzyme, but it is inactive, and we cannot produce uricase. Uricase converts uric acid into allantoin, which is water-soluble and can be excreted through the urine.
Major indications	Severe tophaceous gout or refractory gout.
Other uses	
Contraindications	**Contraindicated with G6PD deficiency.** All patients must be screened prior to initiation.
Side effects	<ul><li>80% chance of causing an acute gouty flare due to rapid lowering of uric acid level within 24 hours.</li><li>Hemolytic anemia and methemoglobinemia in patients with G6PD deficiency.</li><li>Infusion reactions, anaphylaxis.</li></ul>
Lab monitoring	All patients should have serum uric acid level checked before each infusion after the initial dose. A uric acid level > 6 mg/dL on more than two separate occasions portends the development of anti-pegloticase antibodies and loss of efficacy of the medication. Patients who have developed antibodies can have infusion reactions including anaphylaxis, and thus the infusion should not be given if this occurs. For this reason, patients should not receive other uric acid lowering medications because the uric acid level cannot be monitored.
Dose/route/frequency	IV 8 mg/mL infusion every 2 weeks.
Drug interactions	Do not use with other biologics. Do not use with other urate-lower therapies.
Pregnancy category	Limited data.
Patient education	Counsel patients on the high risk of acute gout flares with receiving infusions.
Other notes	*New research shows that CellCept can be used to prevent the development of anti-pegloticase antibodies. [Khanna et al. Reducing Immunogenicity of Pegloticase with Concomitant Use of Mycophenolate Mofetil. Arthritis & Rheumatology, August 2021].

Lesinurad (Zurampic)

Classification	Anti-hyperuricemic agent
Mechanism of action	Inhibits the urate transporter, **URAT1**, which is responsible for the majority of the renal reabsorption of uric acid. Also inhibits organic anion transporter 4 (**OAT4**), a uric acid transporter associated with diuretic-induced hyperuricemia.
Major indications	Given in combination with a xanthine oxidase inhibitor (usually allopurinol) in patients with gout who have not achieved target serum uric acid levels with a xanthine oxidase inhibitor alone.
Other uses	
Contraindications	Avoid with renal insufficiency, CrCl < 45 mL/min. Tumor lysis syndrome or Lesch-Nyhan syndrome.
Side effects	<ul><li>Headaches</li><li>GERD</li><li>Acute renal failure (black box warning)</li><li>Nephrolithiasis</li><li>Cardiovascular events such as MI or stroke</li></ul>
Lab monitoring	Periodic BMP to monitor renal function.
Dose/route/frequency	200 mg PO tablet once daily.
Drug interactions	CYP 2C9 substrates. Makes hormonal contraception less effective.
Pregnancy category	Limited data.
Patient education	Take at the same time of day as taking a xanthine oxidase inhibitor. Stay well-hydrated.
Other notes	

CHAPTER 7

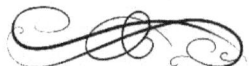

Glucocorticoids

The following glucocorticoid doses are equivalent:

- Prednisone 5 mg
- Prednisolone 5 mg
- Solu-Medrol 4 mg
- Solu-Cortef (Cortisol) 20 mg
- Decadron (Dexamethasone) 0.75 mg

<u>Fluorinated</u>, less soluble steroids have greater potency and last longer.

Prednisone

Classification	Non-fluorinated glucocorticoid
Mechanism of action	Anti-inflammatory effects through multiple mechanisms on both a genomic and non-genomic level. Binds and blocks promoter sites of pro-inflammatory cytokine genes, inhibits production of pro-inflammatory transcription factors, and recruits transcription factors responsible for anti-inflammatory molecules. Binds to glucocorticoid receptors on lymphocytes and monocytes lead to anti-inflammatory effects, and release of inhibitory proteins such as Src.
Major indications	A variety of autoimmune and inflammatory conditions.
Other uses	
Contraindications	
Side effects	<ul><li>Increased risk for infections, especially opportunistic.</li><li>Worsening glucose intolerance and diabetes mellitus.</li><li>Osteoporosis.</li><li>GI upset and peptic ulcer disease, especially when used with NSAIDs.</li><li>Worsening hypertension and cardiovascular disease.</li><li>Steroid-induced psychosis.</li><li>Insomnia, mood changes.</li><li>Cushing syndrome.</li><li>Adrenal insufficiency and suppressed HPA axis.</li><li>Avascular necrosis.</li><li>Cataracts, glaucoma.</li><li>Easy bruising, delayed wound repair.</li><li>Weight gain.</li><li>Muscle weakness and atrophy.</li><li>Acne.</li></ul>
Lab monitoring	No specific guidelines.
Dose/route/frequency	<ul><li>Low dose: < 7.5 mg per day.</li><li>Medium dose: 7.5 to 40 mg per day.</li><li>High dose: > 40 mg per day to 100 mg per day.</li><li>Very high dose: > 100 mg per day.</li></ul>
Drug interactions	Mifepristone.
Pregnancy category	C (immediate release) or D (delayed release). Drug may cause fetal harm and decreased birth weight; maternal corticosteroid use during first trimester increases incidence of cleft lip with or without cleft palate.
Patient education	
Other notes	Requires liver metabolism to active metabolite.

Prednisolone (Medrol)

Classification	Non-fluorinated glucocorticoid
Mechanism of action	Anti-inflammatory effects through multiple mechanisms on both a genomic and non-genomic level. Binds and blocks promoter sites of pro-inflammatory cytokine genes, inhibits production of pro-inflammatory transcription factors, and recruits transcription factors responsible for anti-inflammatory molecules. Binds to glucocorticoid receptors on lymphocytes and monocytes lead to anti-inflammatory effects, and release of inhibitory proteins such as Src.
Major indications	A variety of autoimmune and inflammatory conditions.
Other uses	Allergic dermatitis.
Contraindications	
Side effects	<ul><li>Increased risk for infections, especially opportunistic.</li><li>Worsening glucose intolerance and diabetes mellitus.</li><li>Osteoporosis.</li><li>GI upset and peptic ulcer disease, especially when used with NSAIDs.</li><li>Worsening hypertension and cardiovascular disease.</li><li>Steroid-induced psychosis.</li><li>Insomnia, mood changes.</li><li>Cushing syndrome.</li><li>Adrenal insufficiency and suppressed HPA axis.</li><li>Avascular necrosis.</li><li>Cataracts, glaucoma.</li><li>Easy bruising and delayed wound repair.</li><li>Weight gain, acne.</li><li>Muscle weakness and atrophy.</li></ul>
Lab monitoring	No specific guidelines.
Dose/route/frequency	5, 10, 15, and 30 mg tablets.
Drug interactions	Mifepristone
Pregnancy category	Limited data. Prednisolone should be used during pregnancy only if potential benefit justifies potential risk to fetus.
Patient education	
Other notes	**Does <u>not</u> require the liver to metabolize the drug to its active metabolite** (compared to prednisone, which does).

Methylprednisolone (Solu-Medrol)

Classification	Non-fluorinated glucocorticoid
Mechanism of action	Anti-inflammatory effects through multiple mechanisms on both a genomic and non-genomic level. Binds and blocks promoter sites of pro-inflammatory cytokine genes, inhibits production of pro-inflammatory transcription factors, and recruits transcription factors responsible for anti-inflammatory molecules. Binds to glucocorticoid receptors on lymphocytes and monocytes lead to anti-inflammatory effects, and release of inhibitory proteins such as Src. High dose "pulse" steroids also interfere with calcium and sodium cycling across cell membranes, which exerts anti-inflammatory effects within hours.
Major indications	A variety of autoimmune and inflammatory conditions.
Other uses	
Contraindications	
Side effects	<ul><li>Increased risk for infections, especially opportunistic.</li><li>Worsening glucose intolerance and diabetes mellitus.</li><li>Osteoporosis.</li><li>GI upset and peptic ulcer disease, especially when used with NSAIDs.</li><li>Worsening hypertension and cardiovascular disease.</li><li>Steroid-induced psychosis.</li><li>Insomnia, mood changes.</li><li>Cushing syndrome.</li><li>Adrenal insufficiency and suppressed HPA axis.</li><li>Avascular necrosis.</li><li>Cataracts, glaucoma.</li><li>Easy bruising and delayed wound repair.</li><li>Weight gain.</li><li>Muscle weakness and atrophy.</li><li>Acne.</li></ul>
Lab monitoring	
Dose/route/frequency	Tablets or IV suspension available.
Drug interactions	Mifepristone.
Pregnancy category	C
Patient education	
Other notes	Methylprednisolone acetate is Depo-Medrol, suitable for joint injections.

Dexamethasone (Decadron)

Classification	**Fluorinated** glucocorticoid (higher potency)
Mechanism of action	Anti-inflammatory effects through multiple mechanisms on both a genomic and non-genomic level. Binds and blocks promoter sites of pro-inflammatory cytokine genes, inhibits production of pro-inflammatory transcription factors, and recruits transcription factors responsible for anti-inflammatory molecules. Binds to glucocorticoid receptors on lymphocytes and monocytes lead to anti-inflammatory effects, and release of inhibitory proteins such as Src. High dose "pulse" steroids also interfere with calcium and sodium cycling across cell membranes, which exerts anti-inflammatory effects within hours.
Major indications	A variety of autoimmune and inflammatory conditions.
Other uses	
Contraindications	
Side effects	<ul><li>Increased risk for infections, especially opportunistic.</li><li>Worsening glucose intolerance and diabetes mellitus.</li><li>Osteoporosis.</li><li>GI upset and peptic ulcer disease, especially when used with NSAIDs.</li><li>Worsening hypertension and cardiovascular disease.</li><li>Steroid-induced psychosis.</li><li>Insomnia, mood changes.</li><li>Cushing syndrome.</li><li>Adrenal insufficiency and suppressed HPA axis.</li><li>Avascular necrosis.</li><li>Cataracts, glaucoma.</li><li>Easy bruising and delayed wound repair.</li><li>Weight gain.</li><li>Muscle weakness and atrophy.</li><li>Acne.</li></ul>
Lab monitoring	
Dose/route/frequency	Tablets or IV suspension available.
Drug interactions	Apixaban, mifepristone, roflumilast.
Pregnancy category	Limited data. Adverse developmental outcomes including orofacial clefts (cleft lip with or without cleft palate), intrauterine growth restriction, and decreased birth weight.
Patient education	
Other notes	

Triamcinolone acetonide (Kenalog)

Classification	**Fluorinated** glucocorticoid
Mechanism of action	Anti-inflammatory effects through multiple mechanisms on both a genomic and non-genomic level. Binds and blocks promoter sites of pro-inflammatory cytokine genes, inhibits production of pro-inflammatory transcription factors, and recruits transcription factors responsible for anti-inflammatory molecules. Binds to glucocorticoid receptors on lymphocytes and monocytes lead to anti-inflammatory effects, and release of inhibitory proteins such as Src.
Major indications	A variety of autoimmune and inflammatory conditions.
Other uses	
Contraindications	
Side effects	<ul><li>Studies have shown accelerated deterioration of joints, increased cartilage breakdown or weakening of tendons with steroid injections.</li><li>Infection.</li><li>Skin hypopigmentation.</li><li>Steroid crystal-induced synovitis (post-injection flare occurring about 6-18 hours after an injection).</li><li>Subcutaneous tissue atrophy.</li><li>Tendon rupture. Never inject Achilles tendon.</li><li>Erythroderma.</li></ul>
Lab monitoring	
Dose/route/frequency	Large joints: 15-40 mg. Small joints/tendon sheath inflammation: 2.5-10 mg.
Drug interactions	Mifepristone.
Pregnancy category	Limited data.
Patient education	
Other notes	

Hydrocortisone (Solu-Cortef)

Classification	Non-fluorinated glucocorticoid
Mechanism of action	Elicits mineralocorticoid activity. Exerts anti-inflammatory effects through multiple mechanisms on both a genomic and non-genomic level. Binds and blocks promoter sites of pro-inflammatory cytokine genes, inhibits production of pro-inflammatory transcription factors, and recruits transcription factors responsible for anti-inflammatory molecules. Binds to glucocorticoid receptors on lymphocytes and monocytes lead to anti-inflammatory effects, and release of inhibitory proteins such as Src.
Major indications	A variety of autoimmune and inflammatory conditions.
Other uses	Stress dose of steroids perioperatively for patients with adrenal suppression.
Contraindications	
Side effects	<ul><li>Increased risk for infections, especially opportunistic.</li><li>Worsening glucose intolerance and diabetes mellitus.</li><li>Osteoporosis.</li><li>GI upset and peptic ulcer disease, especially when used with NSAIDs.</li><li>Worsening hypertension and cardiovascular disease.</li><li>Steroid-induced psychosis.</li><li>Insomnia, mood changes.</li><li>Cushing syndrome.</li><li>Adrenal insufficiency and suppressed HPA axis.</li><li>Avascular necrosis.</li><li>Cataracts, glaucoma.</li><li>Easy bruising and delayed wound repair.</li><li>Weight gain.</li><li>Muscle weakness and atrophy.</li><li>Acne.</li></ul>
Lab monitoring	
Dose/route/frequency	Tablets or IV suspension available.
Drug interactions	Mifepristone.
Pregnancy category	C
Patient education	
Other notes	

Acthar Gel (Repository Corticotropin)

Classification	Extracted ACTH
Mechanism of action	Purified preparation of ACTH extracted from pig pituitary glands. ACTH stimulates the adrenal cortex gland to secrete cortisol, corticosterone, and aldosterone. Melanocortin receptor activation on macrophages augment anti-inflammatory responses. Half-life 15 minutes.
Major indications	FDA-approved for a variety of autoimmune diseases, including SLE, dermatomyositis, polymyositis, multiple sclerosis exacerbation, sarcoidosis, inflammatory eye disease.
Other uses	Infantile spasms (rare diagnosis).
Contraindications	
Side effects	<ul><li>Edema</li><li>Hypertension</li><li>Psychosis</li><li>Elevated blood glucose</li><li>Peptic ulcer disease</li><li>Muscle weakness</li><li>Hypersensitivity</li><li>Glaucoma</li><li>Thromboembolism</li><li>Pancreatitis</li><li>Worsening of congestive heart failure</li><li>Cushing's syndrome</li></ul>
Lab monitoring	
Dose/route/frequency	80 unit subcutaneous injection daily or twice per week.
Drug interactions	Amphotericin, testosterone.
Pregnancy category	C
Patient education	
Other notes	Levine, Todd. Treating refractory dermatomyositis or polymyositis with adrenocorticotropic hormone gel: a retrospective case series. Drug Design, Development and Therapy, 2012: 6(133-139).

CHAPTER 8

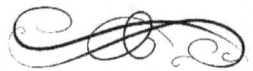

NSAIDs

NSAIDs work through inhibition of COX and decreasing prostaglandin production. They have a number of other effects including inhibition of platelets, lipoxygenase products, superoxides, neutrophil aggregation, cytokine production, and proteoglycan degradation.

COX-1 inhibition: decrease thromboxane production and inhibit platelet activation and clotting.

- Stomach
- Intestine
- Kidney
- Platelets

COX-2 inhibition: reduce inflammation, as well as effects on vascular and thrombotic regulation.

- Kidney
- Brain
- Bone
- Endothelium

COX-3: mostly found in brain tissue in mammals such as dogs, but has very low levels of expression in humans.

Ibuprofen (Advil)

Classification	NSAID – COX nonspecific
Mechanism of action	NSAIDs work through inhibition of COX and decreasing prostaglandin production. They have a number of other effects including inhibition of platelets, lipoxygenase products, superoxides, neutrophil aggregation, cytokine production, and proteoglycan degradation.
Major indications	Analgesia, antipyretic, anti-inflammatory.
Other uses	
Contraindications	See below.
Side effects	<ul><li>Hypersensitivity reaction. Samter's triad – asthma, nasal polyps, and NSAID sensitivity.</li><li>GI side effects: dyspepsia, GERD, gastritis, peptic ulcers, esophagitis.</li><li>Renal side effects: nephrotoxicity, papillary necrosis, interstitial nephritis.</li><li>Increased sodium retention and blood volume – can worsen hypertension and congestive heart failure.</li><li>Increased risk of MI, stroke, and thromboembolism.</li><li>Transaminitis, cholestasis.</li><li>Impaired healing from fractures (controversial).</li><li>Case reports of infertility while taking NSAIDs.</li></ul>
Lab monitoring	CBC and CMP periodically.
Dose/route/frequency	400 to 800 mg PO TID to QID.
Drug interactions	Warfarin, apixaban, diuretics, hypertension medications, phenytoin, lithium, digoxin, aminoglycosides, methotrexate, antacids, probenecid, cholestyramine.
Pregnancy category	May cause premature closure of ductus arteriosus; avoid during 1st and 3rd trimesters.
Patient education	
Other notes	Taking a PPI with NSAID therapy may mitigate GI side effects.

Naproxen (Aleve or Naprosyn)

Classification	NSAID – COX nonspecific
Mechanism of action	NSAIDs work through inhibition of COX and decreasing prostaglandin production. They have a number of other effects including inhibition of platelets, lipoxygenase products, superoxides, neutrophil aggregation, cytokine production, and proteoglycan degradation.
Major indications	Analgesia, antipyresis, anti-inflammatory.
Other uses	
Contraindications	See below.
Side effects	<ul><li>Hypersensitivity reaction. Samter's triad – asthma, nasal polyps, and NSAID sensitivity.</li><li>GI side effects: dyspepsia, GERD, gastritis, peptic ulcers, esophagitis.</li><li>Renal side effects: nephrotoxicity, papillary necrosis, interstitial nephritis.</li><li>Increased sodium retention and blood volume – can worsen hypertension and congestive heart failure.</li><li>Increased risk of MI, stroke, and thromboembolism.</li><li>Transaminitis, cholestasis.</li><li>Impaired healing from fractures (controversial).</li><li>Case reports of infertility while taking NSAIDs.</li></ul>
Lab monitoring	CBC and CMP periodically.
Dose/route/frequency	250 to 500 mg PO BID.
Drug interactions	ACE inhibitors, blood thinners.
Pregnancy category	Limited data. May cause premature closure of ductus arteriosus; avoid during 1st and 3rd trimesters.
Patient education	
Other notes	Taking a PPI with NSAID therapy may mitigate GI side effects.

Indomethacin (Indocin)

Classification	NSAID – COX nonspecific
Mechanism of action	NSAIDs work through inhibition of COX and decreasing prostaglandin production. They have a number of other effects including inhibition of platelets, lipoxygenase products, superoxides, neutrophil aggregation, cytokine production, and proteoglycan degradation.
Major indications	Gout, spondyloarthropathies. Analgesia, antipyresis, anti-inflammatory.
Other uses	
Contraindications	See below.
Side effects	<ul><li>Hypersensitivity reaction. Samter's triad – asthma, nasal polyps, and NSAID sensitivity.</li><li>GI side effects: dyspepsia, GERD, gastritis, peptic ulcers, esophagitis.</li><li>Renal side effects: nephrotoxicity, papillary necrosis, interstitial nephritis.</li><li>Increased sodium retention and blood volume – can worsen hypertension and congestive heart failure.</li><li>Increased risk of MI, stroke, and thromboembolism.</li><li>Transaminitis, cholestasis.</li><li>Impaired healing from fractures (controversial).</li><li>Case reports of infertility while taking NSAIDs.</li></ul>
Lab monitoring	CBC and CMP periodically.
Dose/route/frequency	25 mg PO TID to QID. 50 mg PO TID. 75 mg slow-release PO BID.
Drug interactions	ACE inhibitors, blood thinners.
Pregnancy category	C
Patient education	
Other notes	Taking a PPI with NSAID therapy may mitigate GI side effects.

Etodolac (Lodine)

Classification	NSAID – COX-2 preferential
Mechanism of action	NSAIDs work through inhibition of COX and decreasing prostaglandin production. They have a number of other effects including inhibition of platelets, lipoxygenase products, superoxides, neutrophil aggregation, cytokine production, and proteoglycan degradation.
Major indications	Analgesia, antipyresis, anti-inflammatory.
Other uses	
Contraindications	See below.
Side effects	<ul><li>Hypersensitivity reaction. Samter's triad – asthma, nasal polyps, and NSAID sensitivity.</li><li>GI side effects: dyspepsia, GERD, gastritis, peptic ulcers, esophagitis.</li><li>Renal side effects: nephrotoxicity, papillary necrosis, interstitial nephritis.</li><li>Increased sodium retention and blood volume – can worsen hypertension and congestive heart failure.</li><li>Increased risk of MI, stroke, and thromboembolism.</li><li>Transaminitis, cholestasis.</li><li>Impaired healing from fractures (controversial).</li><li>Case reports of infertility while taking NSAIDs.</li></ul>
Lab monitoring	CBC and CMP periodically.
Dose/route/frequency	200 mg oral tablet TID to QID. 400 mg TID.
Drug interactions	ACE inhibitors, blood thinners.
Pregnancy category	C
Patient education	
Other notes	Taking a PPI with NSAID therapy may mitigate GI side effects.

Diclofenac sodium (Voltaren)

Classification	NSAID – COX-2 preferential
Mechanism of action	NSAIDs work through inhibition of COX and decreasing prostaglandin production. They have a number of other effects including inhibition of platelets, lipoxygenase products, superoxides, neutrophil aggregation, cytokine production, and proteoglycan degradation.
Major indications	Analgesia, antipyresis, anti-inflammatory.
Other uses	
Contraindications	See below.
Side effects	<ul><li>Hypersensitivity reaction. Samter's triad – asthma, nasal polyps, and NSAID sensitivity.</li><li>GI side effects: dyspepsia, GERD, gastritis, peptic ulcers, esophagitis.</li><li>Renal side effects: nephrotoxicity, papillary necrosis, interstitial nephritis.</li><li>Increased sodium retention and blood volume – can worsen hypertension and congestive heart failure.</li><li>Increased risk of MI, stroke, and thromboembolism.</li><li>Transaminitis, cholestasis.</li><li>Impaired healing from fractures (controversial).</li><li>Case reports of infertility while taking NSAIDs.</li></ul>
Lab monitoring	CBC and CMP periodically.
Dose/route/frequency	25-50 mg oral tablet QD to TID. 75 mg oral tablet BID. Other preparations:<ul><li>Diclofenac 1% topical gel (Voltaren topical, now OTC).</li><li>Diclofenac 2% topical gel (Pennsaid) – noted to have 6.6% systemic absorption.</li><li>Diclofenac topical patch (Flector).</li></ul>
Drug interactions	ACE inhibitors, blood thinners.
Pregnancy category	Not defined. May cause premature closure of ductus arteriosus; avoid during 1st and 3rd trimesters.
Patient education	
Other notes	Taking a PPI with NSAID therapy may mitigate GI side effects.

Nabumetone (Relafen)

Classification	NSAID – COX-2 preferential
Mechanism of action	NSAIDs work through inhibition of COX and decreasing prostaglandin production. They have a number of other effects including inhibition of platelets, lipoxygenase products, superoxides, neutrophil aggregation, cytokine production, and proteoglycan degradation.
Major indications	Analgesia, antipyresis, anti-inflammatory.
Other uses	
Contraindications	See below.
Side effects	<ul><li>Hypersensitivity reaction. Samter's triad – asthma, nasal polyps, and NSAID sensitivity.</li><li>GI side effects: dyspepsia, GERD, gastritis, peptic ulcers, esophagitis.</li><li>Renal side effects: nephrotoxicity, papillary necrosis, interstitial nephritis.</li><li>Increased sodium retention and blood volume – can worsen hypertension and congestive heart failure.</li><li>Increased risk of MI, stroke, and thromboembolism.</li><li>Transaminitis, cholestasis.</li><li>Impaired healing from fractures (controversial).</li><li>Case reports of infertility while taking NSAIDs.</li></ul>
Lab monitoring	CBC and CMP periodically.
Dose/route/frequency	500 to 1000 mg PO BID. 1000 to 2000 mg daily.
Drug interactions	ACE inhibitors, blood thinners.
Pregnancy category	C or D
Patient education	
Other notes	Taking a PPI with NSAID therapy may mitigate GI side effects.

Meloxicam (Mobic)

Classification	NSAID – COX-2 preferential
Mechanism of action	NSAIDs work through inhibition of COX and decreasing prostaglandin production. They have a number of other effects including inhibition of platelets, lipoxygenase products, superoxides, neutrophil aggregation, cytokine production, and proteoglycan degradation.
Major indications	Analgesia, antipyresis, anti-inflammatory.
Other uses	
Contraindications	See below.
Side effects	<ul><li>Hypersensitivity reaction. Samter's triad – asthma, nasal polyps, and NSAID sensitivity.</li><li>GI side effects: dyspepsia, GERD, gastritis, peptic ulcers, esophagitis.</li><li>Renal side effects: nephrotoxicity, papillary necrosis, interstitial nephritis.</li><li>Increased sodium retention and blood volume – can worsen hypertension and congestive heart failure.</li><li>Increased risk of MI, stroke, and thromboembolism.</li><li>Transaminitis, cholestasis.</li><li>Impaired healing from fractures (controversial).</li><li>Case reports of infertility while taking NSAIDs.</li></ul>
Lab monitoring	CBC and CMP periodically.
Dose/route/frequency	7.5 to 15 mg PO daily.
Drug interactions	ACE inhibitors, blood thinners, sodium polystyrene sulfonate.
Pregnancy category	C or D
Patient education	
Other notes	Taking a PPI with NSAID therapy may mitigate GI side effects.

Celecoxib (Celebrex)

Classification	NSAID – **COX-2 specific**
Mechanism of action	NSAIDs work through inhibition of COX and decreasing prostaglandin production. They have a number of other effects including inhibition of platelets, lipoxygenase products, superoxides, neutrophil aggregation, cytokine production, and proteoglycan degradation.
Major indications	Analgesia, antipyresis, anti-inflammatory.
Other uses	
Contraindications	See below.
Side effects	<ul><li>**COX-2 selective inhibitors have 50-66% reduced rate of GI complications compared to nonselective inhibitors.**</li><li>Hypersensitivity reaction. Samter's triad – asthma, nasal polyps, and NSAID sensitivity.</li><li>Renal side effects: nephrotoxicity, papillary necrosis, interstitial nephritis.</li><li>Increased sodium retention and blood volume – can worsen hypertension and congestive heart failure.</li><li>Increased risk of MI, stroke, and thromboembolism.</li><li>Transaminitis, cholestasis.</li><li>Impaired healing from fractures (controversial).</li><li>Case reports of infertility while taking NSAIDs.</li></ul>
Lab monitoring	CBC and CMP periodically.
Dose/route/frequency	100 to 200 mg PO once or twice daily.
Drug interactions	ACE inhibitors, blood thinners.
Pregnancy category	C or D
Patient education	
Other notes	

Low dose aspirin

Classification	COX-1 specific
Mechanism of action	Decreases thromboxane production and inhibit platelet activation and clotting.
Major indications	The only COX inhibitor with proven cardioprotective effects.
Other uses	Antiphospholipid antibody syndrome when other anticoagulants are contraindicated.
Contraindications	See below.
Side effects	<ul><li>Hypersensitivity reaction. Samter's triad – asthma, nasal polyps, and aspirin sensitivity.</li><li>GI side effects: dyspepsia, GERD, gastritis, peptic ulcers, esophagitis.</li><li>Renal side effects: nephrotoxicity, papillary necrosis, interstitial nephritis.</li></ul>
Lab monitoring	CBC and CMP periodically.
Dose/route/frequency	81 mg oral tablet once daily.
Drug interactions	Concurrent use of aspirin and NSAIDs increases risk of GI toxicity. Low dose aspirin should be taken more than 2 hours before an NSAID in patients who have to take both medications.
Pregnancy category	Not defined. Low dose aspirin has been used for prevention of preeclampsia in certain situations.
Patient education	
Other notes	

CHAPTER 9

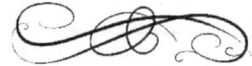

Osteoporosis Medications

Indications to start pharmacologic therapy for osteoporosis:

1. History of vertebral or hip fragility fractures (defined as a fracture resulting from a fall at standing height or less).

2. T score < -2.5.

3. Patients with osteopenia and the FRAX tool indicating a 10-year risk of > 3% for hip fracture or > 20% for other major osteoporosis fractures.

Alendronate (Fosamax)

Classification	Antiresorptive agent – bisphosphonate
Mechanism of action	Inhibits osteoclast-mediated bone resorption. Acts on osteoclasts by binding and blocking the **farnesyl diphosphate synthase (FPPS)** enzyme. This disrupts prenylation of small proteins and interferes with lipid modification of the osteoclast cell membrane and cytoskeleton. Osteoclast apoptosis results. Bone formation exceeds bone resorption and bone mass increases.
Major indications	Osteoporosis.
Other uses	Paget disease.
Contraindications	Esophageal stricture, Schatzki ring, achalasia, dysmotility, or inability to sit upright. Contraindicated in renal insufficiency with CrCl < 30-35 mL/min.
Side effects	<ul><li>Esophagitis and GI pain.</li><li>Osteonecrosis of the jaw, presenting as persistently exposed bone following an invasive dental procedure. All invasive dental work should be done before starting a bisphosphonate, if possible.</li><li>Atypical femoral fractures, usually occurs after taking a bisphosphonate for more than 5 years. Keep this in mind for patients with unexplained thigh pain. A drug holiday for 1-2 years after 5 years of bisphosphonate use decreases the risk for atypical fractures by 70%.</li><li>Rarely can cause ocular symptoms including uveitis, keratitis, optic neuritis, and orbital swelling.</li><li>Hypocalcemia.</li></ul>
Lab monitoring	Make sure 25-OH-vitamin D level is > 20-30 before starting therapy.
Dose/route/frequency	Osteoporosis: 70 mg oral tablet once per week. Paget disease: 40 mg oral tablet per day for 6 months.
Drug interactions	No significant interactions identified.
Pregnancy category	Limited data. Avoid with pregnancy – causes unknown effects on the developing fetal skeleton.
Patient education	Medication should be taken first thing each morning on an empty stomach with a full glass of water. Patient should remain upright and take nothing by mouth for 30-60 minutes after ingestion. Do not take with coffee, juice, or mineral water. Encourage good oral hygiene and regular dental care as prevention against jaw osteonecrosis.
Other notes	

Risedronate (Actonel, Atelvia)

Classification	Antiresorptive agent – bisphosphonate
Mechanism of action	Inhibits osteoclast-mediated bone resorption. Acts on osteoclasts by binding and blocking the **farnesyl diphosphate synthase (FPPS)** enzyme. This disrupts prenylation of small proteins and interferes with lipid modification of the osteoclast cell membrane and cytoskeleton. Osteoclast apoptosis results. Bone formation exceeds bone resorption and bone mass increases.
Major indications	Osteoporosis.
Other uses	Paget disease.
Contraindications	Esophageal stricture, Schatzki ring, achalasia, dysmotility, or inability to sit upright. Contraindicated in renal insufficiency with CrCl < 30-35 mL/min.
Side effects	<ul><li>Esophagitis and GI pain.</li><li>Osteonecrosis of the jaw, presenting as persistently exposed bone following an invasive dental procedure. All invasive dental work should be done before starting a bisphosphonate, if possible.</li><li>Atypical femoral fractures, usually occurs after taking a bisphosphonate for more than 5 years. Keep this in mind for patients with unexplained thigh pain. A drug holiday for 1-2 years after 5 years of bisphosphonate use decreases the risk for atypical fractures by 70%.</li><li>Rarely can cause ocular symptoms including uveitis, keratitis, optic neuritis, and orbital swelling.</li><li>Hypocalcemia.</li></ul>
Lab monitoring	Make sure 25-OH-vtamin D level is > 20-30 before starting therapy.
Dose/route/frequency	Osteoporosis: 35 mg tablet once per week or 150 mg once monthly. Paget disease: 30 mg tablet once per day for 2 months.
Drug interactions	No significant interactions identified.
Pregnancy category	Limited data. Avoid with pregnancy – causes unknown effects on the developing fetal skeleton.
Patient education	Medication should be taken first thing each morning on an empty stomach with a full glass of water. Patient should remain upright and take nothing by mouth for 30-60 minutes after ingestion. Do not take with coffee, juice, or mineral water. Encourage good oral hygiene and regular dental care as prevention against jaw osteonecrosis.
Other notes	

Ibandronate (Boniva)

Classification	Antiresorptive agent – Bisphosphonate
Mechanism of action	Inhibits osteoclast-mediated bone resorption. Acts on osteoclasts by binding and blocking the **farnesyl diphosphate synthase (FPPS)** enzyme. This disrupts prenylation of small proteins and interferes with lipid modification of the osteoclast cell membrane and cytoskeleton. Osteoclast apoptosis results. Bone formation exceeds bone resorption and bone mass increases.
Major indications	Osteoporosis.
Other uses	Paget disease.
Contraindications	Esophageal stricture, Schatzki ring, achalasia, dysmotility, or inability to sit upright. Contraindicated in renal insufficiency with CrCl < 30-35 mL/min.
Side effects	<ul><li>Esophagitis and GI pain.</li><li>Osteonecrosis of the jaw, presenting as persistently exposed bone following an invasive dental procedure. All invasive dental work should be done before starting a bisphosphonate, if possible.</li><li>Atypical femoral fractures, usually occurs after taking a bisphosphonate for more than 5 years. Keep this in mind for patients with unexplained thigh pain. A drug holiday for 1-2 years after 5 years of bisphosphonate use decreases the risk for atypical fractures by 70%.</li><li>Rarely can cause ocular symptoms including uveitis, keratitis, optic neuritis, and orbital swelling.</li><li>Hypocalcemia.</li><li>Back pain.</li></ul>
Lab monitoring	Make sure 25-OH-vtamin D level is > 20-30 before starting therapy.
Dose/route/frequency	150 mg oral tablet once per month. IV 3 mg infusion once every 3 months.
Drug interactions	
Pregnancy category	Limited data. Avoid with pregnancy – causes unknown effects on the developing fetal skeleton.
Patient education	Medication should be taken first thing each morning on an empty stomach with a full glass of water. Patient should remain upright and take nothing by mouth for 30-60 minutes after ingestion. Do not take with coffee, juice, or mineral water. Encourage good oral hygiene and regular dental care as prevention against jaw osteonecrosis.
Other notes	

Zoledronic acid (Reclast, Zometa)

Classification	Antiresorptive agent – Bisphosphonate
Mechanism of action	Inhibits osteoclast-mediated bone resorption. Acts on osteoclasts by binding and blocking the **farnesyl diphosphate synthase (FPPS)** enzyme. This disrupts prenylation of small proteins and interferes with lipid modification of the osteoclast cell membrane and cytoskeleton. Osteoclast apoptosis results. Bone formation exceeds bone resorption and bone mass increases.
Major indications	Osteoporosis.
Other uses	Paget disease.
Contraindications	Contraindicated in renal insufficiency with CrCl < 30-35 mL/min.
Side effects	<ul><li>Infusions can cause flu-like symptoms and bone pain.</li><li>Osteonecrosis of the jaw, presenting as persistently exposed bone following an invasive dental procedure. All invasive dental work should be done before starting a bisphosphonate, if possible.</li><li>Atypical femoral fractures, usually occurs after taking a bisphosphonate for more than 5 years. Keep this in mind for patients with unexplained thigh pain. A drug holiday for 3 years after 3 years of zoledronic acid decreases the risk for atypical fractures by 70%.</li><li>Rarely can cause ocular symptoms including uveitis, keratitis, optic neuritis, and orbital swelling.</li></ul>
Lab monitoring	Make sure 25-OH-vtamin D level is > 20-30 before starting therapy.
Dose/route/frequency	IV 5 mg infusion once per year, which may be better for compliance.
Drug interactions	
Pregnancy category	Limited data. Avoid with pregnancy – causes unknown effects on the developing fetal skeleton.
Patient education	
Other notes	The best choice for patients with contraindications to taking oral bisphosphonates (such as GERD or esophageal strictures) or to increase compliance.

Denosumab (Prolia)

Classification	Biologic, antiresorptive agent
Mechanism of action	Monoclonal antibody that targets **RANKL**. Binds to RANKL and inhibits its binding to RANK receptor, thereby preventing **osteoclast** formation. This results in decreased bone resorption and increases bone mass in osteoporosis.
Major indications	Osteoporosis.
Other uses	
Contraindications	Pregnancy.
Side effects	<ul><li>Osteonecrosis of jaw</li><li>Atypical fractures</li><li>Hypocalcemia, especially with CKD</li><li>Back pain</li><li>Hypersensitivity or injection reaction</li></ul>
Lab monitoring	
Dose/route/frequency	60 mg subcutaneous injection once every 6 months.
Drug interactions	
Pregnancy category	Contraindicated in pregnancy. Women need reliable contraception. Avoid attempting conception for at least 5 months after the last dose of Denosumab.
Patient education	
Other notes	Can be used in patients with CKD stage 4.

Raloxifene (Evista)

Classification	Antiresorptive agent – SERM
Mechanism of action	Selective estrogen receptor modulators function as estrogen agonists in bone and breast tissue. Reduces risk of spine/vertebral fractures. Has **not** been shown to reduce the risk of a hip fracture.
Major indications	Postmenopausal osteoporosis.
Other uses	Postmenopausal hot flashes. Also reduces risk of breast cancer.
Contraindications	History of DVT/PE, stroke.
Side effects	<ul><li>**Thromboembolic disease**, especially in smokers.</li><li>**Increased risk of strokes.**</li><li>Hot flashes, flu-like malaise.</li><li>Leg cramps, joint pain.</li></ul>
Lab monitoring	
Dose/route/frequency	60 mg oral tablet once daily.
Drug interactions	Ospemifene, cholestyramine.
Pregnancy category	X
Patient education	
Other notes	The ideal patient to receive raloxifene is a patient with osteoporosis as well as a personal or family history of breast cancer.

Calcitonin (Miacalcin)

Classification	Antiresorptive agent
Mechanism of action	Inhibits osteoclastic bone resorption, decreases serum calcium, and increases renal excretion of phosphate, calcium, sodium magnesium and potassium by decreasing tubular reabsorption.
Major indications	Osteoporosis.
Other uses	Paget disease, hypercalcemia.
Contraindications	
Side effects	<ul><li>Rhinitis</li><li>Arthralgia, back pain</li><li>Epistaxis</li><li>Injection site reaction or hypersensitivity</li><li>Nausea</li><li>Headache</li><li>Flushing</li></ul>
Lab monitoring	
Dose/route/frequency	200 units nasal mist once daily. 100 unit subcutaneous injection once daily.
Drug interactions	
Pregnancy category	Limited data.
Patient education	
Other notes	

Teriparatide (Forteo)

Classification	Anabolic agent
Mechanism of action	Amino acid fragment of intact PTH that can bind to and activate PTH receptors on osteoblasts and osteoblast precursors. Stimulates osteoblast function, increases calcium absorption, and increases renal tubular reabsorption of calcium. Intermittent daily pulses of exogenous PTH stimulates osteoblast differentiation, proliferation, and survival, resulting in increased bone mass.
Major indications	Osteoporosis.
Other uses	Hypoparathyroidism.
Contraindications	Patients at risk for osteosarcomas, Paget's disease, unexplained alkaline phosphatase elevation, children with open epiphyses, previous radiation therapy involving the skeleton, skeletal metastases, multiple myeloma.
Side effects	<ul><li>Headache</li><li>Nausea</li><li>Arthralgias</li><li>Orthostasis</li><li>Flushing</li><li>Hypercalcemia</li><li>Hyperuricemia</li><li>Increased risk for osteosarcoma</li></ul>
Lab monitoring	Check PTH and vitamin D level before starting.
Dose/route/frequency	20 μgram subcutaneous injection once daily, usually given for 18-24 months. Do not use for more than 2 years.
Drug interactions	Digoxin.
Pregnancy category	Limited data.
Patient education	
Other notes	After completing treatment with teriparatide, patients should take an antiresorptive agent such as a bisphosphonate to preserve the bone mass that was gained.

Abaloparatide (Tymlos)

Classification	Anabolic agent
Mechanism of action	Synthetic peptide analog of human parathyroid hormone-related protein (hPTHrP) that can bind to and activate PTH receptors on osteoblasts and osteoblast precursors. Stimulates osteoblast function, increases calcium absorption, and increases renal tubular reabsorption of calcium. Intermittent daily pulses of exogenous PTH stimulates osteoblast differentiation, proliferation, and survival, resulting in increased bone mass.
Major indications	Osteoporosis.
Other uses	Hypoparathyroidism.
Contraindications	Patients at risk for osteosarcomas, Paget's disease, unexplained alkaline phosphatase elevation, children with open epiphyses, previous radiation therapy involving the skeleton, skeletal metastases, multiple myeloma.
Side effects	<ul><li>Headache</li><li>Nausea</li><li>Arthralgias</li><li>Orthostasis</li><li>Flushing</li><li>Hypercalcemia</li><li>Hyperuricemia</li><li>Increased risk for osteosarcoma</li></ul>
Lab monitoring	Check PTH and vitamin D level before starting.
Dose/route/frequency	80 μgram subcutaneous injection once daily, usually given for 18-24 months. Do not use for more than 2 years.
Drug interactions	
Pregnancy category	Limited data.
Patient education	
Other notes	

Romosozumab (Evenity)

Classification	Biologic, antiresorptive agent
Mechanism of action	Monoclonal antibody (IgG2) that binds and **inhibits sclerostin**, a regulatory factor in bone metabolism. Sclerostin has been shown to bind LRP5 and LRP6, thereby **inhibiting Wnt signaling.** This prevents Wnt from forming complexes with Frizzled family receptors, preventing accumulation of β-catenin in the cytoplasm and its translocation into the nucleus. **Inhibition of sclerostin** allows increased activation of the canonical Wnt and β-catenin pathway, ultimately increasing bone formation and, to a lesser extent, decreasing bone resorption.
Major indications	Osteoporosis.
Other uses	
Contraindications	History of MI or stroke.
Side effects	<ul><li>May increase the risk of MI, stroke, and cardiovascular death</li><li>Osteonecrosis of the jaw</li><li>Atypical femoral fracture</li><li>Arthralgias</li><li>Headaches</li><li>Injection site reactions or hypersensitivity</li><li>Muscle spasms</li><li>Restless legs</li><li>Paresthesias</li><li>Hypocalcemia</li></ul>
Lab monitoring	
Dose/route/frequency	210 mg subcutaneous injection once per month for 12 months. Supplement with calcium and vitamin D during treatment.
Drug interactions	
Pregnancy category	Limited data.
Patient education	
Other notes	

CHAPTER 10

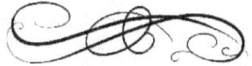

Investigational Drugs

These medications are still being investigated. Some of them are close to FDA approval and may be available in 2024. Others have shown significant adverse effects and may not be approved.

Tanezumab

Classification	Biologic under investigation for osteoarthritis
Mechanism of action	Investigational humanized monoclonal antibody that binds and inhibits **nerve growth factor** (NGF). Disrupts pain signal transmission to the spinal cord and brain.
FDA approvals	Potentially osteoarthritis.
Other uses	
Contraindications	
Side effects	<ul><li>Rapidly progressive OA.</li><li>Increased rate of total joint replacements in 40-week observation periods.</li><li>Patients with **avascular necrosis** and subchondral fractures were excluded from the most recent study.</li></ul>
Lab monitoring	
Dose/route/frequency	2.5 mg oral tablet at week 1 and 5 mg at week 8.
Drug interactions	
Pregnancy category	
Patient education	
Other notes	

Filgotinib

Classification	JAK inhibitor, pending FDA approval
Mechanism of action	**Selective for JAK1.** Inhibition of JAK intracellular proteins and transduction for a number of cytokine and growth factor receptors. Half-life 3 hours. • Inhibition of JAK1/JAK2 (important for IL-6 and IFN signaling). • Inhibition of JAK1/JAK3 (important for T and B cell signaling). • Prevents phosphorylation and activation of STATs (signal transducers and activators of transcription).
FDA approvals	Likely RA.
Other uses	Possibly Crohn's disease.
Contraindications	May be similar to other JAK inhibitors.
Side effects	• Nausea • Liver enzyme elevation • CK elevation • Thrombocytosis • Herpes zoster infection and other serious infections • Lymphoma and other malignancies • Thromboembolism • GI perforation • Upper respiratory infections • Low blood cell counts
Lab monitoring	May be similar to other JAK inhibitors.
Dose/route/frequency	100 or 200 mg tablets.
Other notes	

Brepocitinib

Classification	Tyrosine kinase 2 (**TYK2**) inhibitor and JAK1 inhibitor pending FDA approval
Mechanism of action	Inhibition of intracellular proteins and transduction for a number of cytokine and growth factor receptors. TYK2 differs from other JAK family subtypes in its cytokine signaling specificity. TYK2 primarily regulates **interferon-α, IL-12, and IL-23**.
FDA approvals	Potentially RA and psoriatic arthritis in phase IIb trials. Phase 3 trials for Dermatomyositis.
Other uses	Selective inhibition of TYK2 could potentially provide pharmacological benefits in the treatment of many diseases such as psoriasis, systemic lupus erythematosus (SLE), inflammatory bowel disease (IBD), cancer, and diabetes.
Contraindications	May be similar to other JAK inhibitors.
Side effects	May be similar to other JAK inhibitors.
Lab monitoring	May be similar to other JAK inhibitors.
Dose/route/frequency	Not yet known.
Other notes	Nogueira M, Puig L, Torres T. JAK Inhibitors for Treatment of Psoriasis: Focus on Selective TYK2 Inhibitors. Drugs. 2020 Mar;80(4):341-352. Vleugels RA, et al; VALOR Investigators. A Phase 3 Trial of Brepocitinib in Dermatomyositis. N Engl J Med. 2026 Mar 28. doi: 10.1056/NEJMoa2503531. Epub ahead of print. PMID: 41910335.

Olokizumab

Classification	Biologic – IL-6 inhibitor under investigation
Mechanism of action	
FDA approvals	Pending – rheumatoid arthritis with inadequate response to methotrexate
Other uses	
Contraindications	Similar to other IL-6 inhibitors
Side effects	Similar to other IL-6 inhibitors
Lab monitoring	
Dose/route/frequency	64 mg subcutaneous injection every 2 or 4 weeks
Other notes	Smolen et al. Olokizumab versus Placebo or Adalimumab in Rheumatoid Arthritis. NEJM 387;8, August 2022.

Nipocalimab

Classification	Biologic under investigation
Mechanism of action	Human IgG1 monoclonal antibody that binds to neonatal Fc receptor (FcRn), resulting in reduction of circulating IgG levels. FcRn prolongs IgG half-life; antagonizing FcRn causes IgG catabolism, resulting in reduced overall IgG and pathogenic autoantibody levels, while avoiding widespread immunosuppression.
FDA approvals	Pending for **Sjogren syndrome**
Other uses	Myasthenia Gravis
Contraindications	Infection, Coadministration with medications that bind to FcRn (eg, immunoglobulin products, monoclonal antibodies, or antibody derivates containing human Fc domain of the IgG subclass) may lower systemic exposures and reduce effectiveness of such medications.
Side effects	Increase in total cholesterol Infusion reactions
Lab monitoring	
Dose/route/frequency	In clinical trials, patients received an infusion given as intravenous nipocalimab 5 mg/kg, intravenous nipocalimab 15 mg/kg, or placebo every 2 weeks for 22 weeks.
Other notes	Noaiseh G, Sivils KL, Campbell K, Idokogi J, Lo KH, Liva SG, Leu JH, Dhatt H, Ma K, Leonardo S, Li H, Hubbard JJ, Gottenberg JE. Efficacy and safety of nipocalimab in patients with moderate-to-severe Sjögren's disease (DAHLIAS): a randomised, phase 2, placebo-controlled, double-blind trial. Lancet. 2025 Nov 22;406(10518):2435-2448.

Ianalumab

Classification	Biologic under investigation
Mechanism of action	**Dual Function:** It combines B-cell depletion (via ADCC) with blocking BAFF-R-mediated signals, essential for B-cell survival and maturation. **Target:** The BAFF receptor (BAFF-R) on B-cells.
FDA approvals	Pending for **Sjogren syndrome**
Other uses	Immune thrombocytopenia (ITP), possibly Lupus (SLE), lupus nephritis
Contraindications	Infection
Side effects	One incidental finding of asymptomatic cytomegalovirus infection (patient was IgM-positive in the study).
Lab monitoring	Unclear.
Dose/route/frequency	In clinical trials, patients received ianalumab 300 mg subcutaneous monthly compared with placebo for 52 weeks.
Other notes	Dörner T, Bowman SJ, Fox R, Mariette X, Papas A, Grader-Beck T, Fisher BA, Barcelos F, De Vita S, Schulze-Koops H, Moots RJ, Junge G, Woznicki J, Sopala M, Avrameas A, Luo WL, Hueber W. Safety and Efficacy of Ianalumab in Patients With Sjögren's Disease: 52-Week Results From a Randomized, Placebo-Controlled, Phase 2b Dose-Ranging Study. Arthritis Rheumatol. 2025 May;77(5):560-570.

Rontalizumab

Classification	Interferon inhibitor under investigation
Mechanism of action	Humanized monoclonal antibody against interferon-alpha. Blockade of interferon signaling inhibits downstream inflammatory and immunological processes, including plasma cell differentiation.
FDA approvals	Pending - moderate to severe SLE.
Other uses	
Contraindications	Active infections.
Side effects	Increased risk of infections such as herpes zoster.
Lab monitoring	
Dose/route/frequency	Not yet known.
Other notes	Kalunian et al. A Phase II study of the efficacy and safety of rontalizumab (rhuMAb interferon-alpha) in patients with systemic lupus erythematosus (ROSE). Annals of Rheumatic Disease, January 2016; 75(1): 196-202.

Sifalimumab

Classification	Interferon inhibitor under investigation
Mechanism of action	Humanized monoclonal antibody against interferon-alpha. Blockade of interferon signaling inhibits downstream inflammatory and immunological processes, including plasma cell differentiation.
FDA approvals	Pending - moderate to severe SLE.
Other uses	
Contraindications	Active infections.
Side effects	Increased risk of infections such as herpes zoster.
Lab monitoring	
Dose/route/frequency	Not yet known.
Other notes	Khamashta et al. Sifalimumab, an anti-interferon-alpha monoclonal antibody, in moderate to severe systemic lupus erythematosus: a randomized, double-blind, placebo-controlled study. Annals of the Rheumatic Diseases 2016; 75: 1909-1916.

Lenabasum

Classification	Novel non-psychoactive cannabinoid
Mechanism of action	Targets **cannabinoid receptor-2**. Lenabasum has been shown to downregulate IL-31, a mediator of itch, and IL-4. Lenabasum also significantly reduced IFN-β protein and mRNA in skin compared to placebo.
FDA approvals	?Potentially pruritus secondary to dermatomyositis or scleroderma.
Other uses	
Contraindications	
Side effects	<ul><li>Dizziness</li><li>Dry mouth</li></ul>
Lab monitoring	
Dose/route/frequency	
Drug interactions	
Pregnancy category	
Patient education	
Other notes	Werth V, Hejazi E, Pena S, Haber J, Okawa J, Feng R, et al. A phase 2 study of safety and efficacy of lenabasum (JBT-101), a cannabinoid receptor type 2 agonist, in refractory skin-predominant dermatomyositis.

CAR T-Cell Therapy

Mechanism of action	CAR T-cell therapy is an emerging, highly promising treatment for severe, refractory lupus (SLE) that involves re-engineering a patient's T-cells to destroy autoreactive B-cells. Early studies show it can lead to drug-free, long-term remission, essentially "resetting" the immune system, with trials indicating significant improvements for patients who failed conventional treatments. T-cells are collected, modified to target CD19 (a protein on B-cells), and infused back to eliminate the B-cells driving the autoimmune attack.
FDA approvals	Lymphoma, certain types of cancers Potentially Lupus, lupus nephritis, scleroderma
Side effects	<ul><li>Cytokine Release Syndrome (CRS): The most common side effect, involving a high-intensity immune response causing fever, chills, nausea, fatigue, tachycardia, and low blood pressure</li><li>Immune Effector Cell-Associated Neurotoxicity Syndrome (ICANS): Affects the nervous system, leading to temporary symptoms like headaches, confusion, agitation, delirium, or difficulty speaking.</li><li>LICATS (Local Immune Effector Cell-Associated Toxicity Syndrome): A recently described phenomenon, occurring particularly in organs previously affected by lupus (e.g., skin rashes, joint pain, or proteinuria). These are typically mild, transient, and self-limiting.</li><li>Infection Risk: Because the therapy involves B-cell depletion and chemotherapy, patients are at risk for infections, requiring close monitoring and preventative treatment.</li><li>Worsening of Underlying Lupus: Temporary exacerbation of lupus symptoms can occur during the initial phase of treatment.</li></ul>
Other notes	Schett G, Mackensen A, Mougiakakos D. CAR T-cell therapy in autoimmune diseases. Lancet. 2023 Nov 25;402(10416):2034-2044. doi: 10.1016/S0140-6736(23)01126-1. Epub 2023 Sep 22. PMID: 37748491. Mackensen A, Müller F, Mougiakakos D, Böltz S, Wilhelm A, Aigner M, Völkl S, Simon D, Kleyer A, Munoz L, Kretschmann S, Kharboutli S, Gary R, Reimann H, Rösler W, Uderhardt S, Bang H, Herrmann M, Ekici AB, Buettner C, Habenicht KM, Winkler TH, Krönke G, Schett G. Anti-CD19 CAR T cell therapy for refractory systemic lupus erythematosus. Nat Med. 2022 Oct;28(10):2124-2132. doi: 10.1038/s41591-022-02017-5.

For updated information on rheumatologic drugs under investigation, visit clinicaltrials.gov.

References

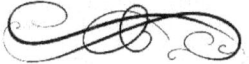

1. West, Sterling and Kolfenbach, Jason. Rheumatology Secrets. Fourth edition, 2019.

2. Bird P., Griffiths H., Tymms K., et al: The Simle study – safety of methotrexate in combination with leflunomide in rheumatoid arthritis. J Rheumatol 2013; 40: pp. 228-235

3. Braun et al., 2008. Braun J., Kastner P., and Flaxenberg P.: Comparison of the clinical efficacy and safety of subcutaneous versus oral administration of methotrexate in patients with active rheumatoid arthritis. Arthritis Rheum 2008; 58: pp. 73-81

4. Cannella and O'Dell, 2017. Cannella A.C., and O'Dell J.R.: Traditional DMARDs: methotrexate, leflunomide, sulfasalazine, hydroxychloroquine, and combination therapies. In Firestein G.S. (eds): Kelley & Firestein's Textbook of Rheumatology, 10th ed. Philadelphia: Elsevier, 2017. pp. 958-982

5. Felson et al., 1995. Felson D.T., Anderson J.J., Boers M., et al: American college of rheumatology preliminary definition for improvement in rheumatoid arthritis. Arthritis Rheum 1995; 38: pp. 727-735

6. Hoekstra et al., 2006. Hoekstra M., Haagsma C., Neef C., et al: Splitting high-dose oral methotrexate improves the bioavailability: a pharmacokinetic study in patients with rheumatoid arthritis. J Rheumatol 2006; 33: pp. 481-485

7. Izmirly et al., 2012. Izmirly P.M., Costedoat-Chalumeau N., Bunyon J.P., et al: Maternal use of hydroxychloroquine is associated with a reduced risk of recurrent anti-SSA/Ro-antibody–associated cardiac manifestations of neonatal lupus. Circulation 2012; 126: pp. 76-82

8. Katz and Russell, 2011. Katz S.J., and Russell A.S.: Re-evaluation of antimalarials in treating rheumatic diseases: re-appreciation and insights into new mechanisms of action. Curr Opin Rheumatol 2011; 23: pp. 278-281

9. Kremer, 2004. Kremer J.: Toward a better understanding of methotrexate. Arthritis Rheum 2004; 50: pp. 1370-1382.

10. Landewe et al., 2002. Landewe R.B.M., Boers M., Verhoeven A.C., et al: COBRA combination therapy in patients with early rheumatoid arthritis: long-term structural benefits of a brief intervention. Arthritis Rheum 2002; 46: pp. 347-356

11. Marmor et al., 2016. Marmor M.F., Kellner U., Lai T.Y., Melles R.B., and Mieler W.F.: Recommendations on screening for chloroquine and hydroxychloroquine retinopathy (2016 Revision). Ophthalmology 2016; 123: pp. 1386-1394

12. Melles and Marmor, 2014. Melles R.B., and Marmor M.F.: The risk of toxic retinopathy in patients on long-term hydroxychloroquine therapy. JAMA Ophthalmol 2014; 132: pp. 1453-1460

13. Moreland et al., 2012. Moreland L.W., O'Dell J.R., Paulus H.E., et al: A randomized comparative effectiveness study of oral triple therapy versus etanercept plus methotrexate in early aggressive rheumatoid arthritis: the treatment of early aggressive rheumatoid arthritis trial. Arthritis Rheum 2012; 64: pp. 2824-2835

14. O'Dell et al., 1996. O'Dell J.R., Haire C., Erikson N., et al: Treatment of rheumatoid arthritis with methotrexate, sulfasalazine, and hydroxychloroquine, or a combination of these medications. N Engl J Med 1996; 334: pp. 1287-1291

15. O'Dell et al., 1997. O'Dell J.R., Haire C.E., Moore G.F., et al: Treatment of early rheumatoid arthritis with minocycline or placebo. Arthritis Rheum 1997; 40: pp. 842-848

16. Plosker and Croom, 2005. Plosker G., and Croom K.: Sulfasalazine: a review of its use in the management of rheumatoid arthritis. Drugs 2005; 65: pp. 1825-1849

17. SinghSaag and Bridges, 2015. Singh J.A., Saag K.G., Bridges S.L., et al: American College of Rheumatology guideline for the treatment of rheumatoid arthritis. Arthritis Care Res 2015; 68: pp. 1-26

18. Smolen et al., 1999. Smolen J., Kalden J.R., Scott D.L., et al: Efficacy and safety of leflunomide compared with placebo and sulphasalazine in active rheumatoid arthritis: a double-blind, randomized, multicentre trial. Lancet 1999; 353: pp. 259-266

19. Smolen et al., 2017. Smolen J.S., Landewe R., Bijlsma J., et al: EULAR recommendations for the management of rheumatoid arthritis with synthetic and biological disease-modifying antirheumatic drugs: 2016 update. Ann Rheum Dis 2017; 76: pp. 960-977

20. Wolfe and Marmor, 2010. Wolfe F., and Marmor M.F.: Rates and predictors of hydroxychloroquine retinal toxicity in patients with rheumatoid arthritis and systemic lupus erythematosus. Arthritis Care Res 2010; 62: pp. 775-784

21. Allem et al., 2019. Allem K.B., and Keating R.M.: Immunosuppressive agents: cyclosporine, cyclophosphamide, azathioprine, mycophenolate mofetil, and tacrolimus. In Hochberg M.C. (eds): Rheumatology, 7th ed. Philadelphia: Elsevier, 2019. pp. 518-526

22. Ballow, 2011. Ballow M.: The IgG molecule as a biological immune response modifier: mechanisms of action of intravenous immune serum globulin in autoimmune and inflammatory disorders. J Allergy Clin Immunol 2011; 127: pp. 315-323

23. Bejarano et al., 2009. Bejarano V., Conaghan P.G., Proudman S.M., et al: Long-term efficacy and toxicity of cyclosporine A in combination with methotrexate in poor prognosis rheumatoid arthritis. Ann Rheum Dis 2009; 68: pp. 761-763

24. Blumenfeld et al., 2000. Blumenfeld Z., Shapiro D., Shteinberg M., et al: Preservation of fertility and ovarian function and minimizing gonadotoxicity in young women with systemic lupus erythematosus treated by chemotherapy. Lupus 2000; 9: pp. 401-405

25. de Jonge et al., 2005. de Jonge M.E., Huitema A.D., Rodenhuis S., et al: Clinical pharmacokinetics of cyclophosphamide. Clin Pharmacokinet 2005; 44: pp. 1135-1164

26. Fields et al., 1998. Fields C.L., Robinson J.W., Roy T.M., et al: Hypersensitivity reaction to azathioprine. South Med J 1998; 91: pp. 471-474

27. Gerbino et al., 2008. Gerbino A.J., Goss C.H., and Molitor J.A.: Effect of mycophenolate mofetil on pulmonary function in scleroderma-associated interstitial lung disease. Chest 2008; 133: pp. 455-460

28. Hatemi et al., 2015. Hatemi G., Melikoglu M., Tunc R., et al: Apremilast for Behcet's syndrome – a phase 2, placebo-controlled study. N Engl J Med 2015; 372: pp. 1510-1518

29. Haubitz et al., 2002. Haubitz M., Bohnenstengel F., Brunkhorst R., et al: Cyclophosphamide pharmacokinetics and dose adjustments in patients with renal insufficiency. Kidney Internat 2002; 61: pp. 1495-1501

30. Majhail et al., 2015. Majhail N.S., Farnia S.H., Carpenter P.A., et al: Indications for autologous and allogeneic hematopoietic cell transplantation: guidelines from the American Society for Blood and Marrow Transplantation. Biol Blood Marrow Transplant 2015; 21: pp. 1863-1869

31. Monach et al., 2010. Monach P.A., Arnold L.M., and Merkel P.A.: Incidence and prevention of bladder toxicity from cyclophosphamide in the treatment of rheumatic diseases. A data driven review. Arthritis Rheum 2010; 62: pp. 9-21

32. Perez et al., 2017. Perez E.E., Orange J.S., Bonilla F., Chinen J., Chinn I.K., Dorsey M., et al: Update on the use of immunoglobulin in human disease: a review of evidence. J Allergy Clin Immunol 2017; 139: pp. S1-S46

33. Reed and Crosbie, 2017. Reed M., and Crosbie D.: Apremilast in the treatment of psoriatic arthritis: a perspective review. Ther Adv Musculoskeletal Dis 2017; 9: pp. 45-53

34. Schedel et al., 2006. Schedel J., Godde A., Schutz E., et al: Impact of thiopurine methyltransferase activity and 6-thioguanine nucleotide concentrations in patients with chronic inflammatory diseases. Ann NY Acad Sci 2006; 1069: pp. 477-491

35. Schwartz et al., 2017. Schwartz D.M., Kanno Y., Villarino A., et al: JAK inhibition as a strategy for immune and inflammatory diseases. Nature Rev Drug Discovery 2017; 16: pp. 843-862

36. Schwartz et al., 2016. Schwartz J., Padmanabhan A., Aqui N., Balogun R.A., Connelly-Smith L., Delaney M., et al: Guidelines on the use of therapeutic apheresis in clinical practice-evidence-based approach from the writing committee of the American Society for Apheresis: the seventh special issue. J Clin Apher 2016; 31: pp. 149-162

37. Smolen et al., 2017. Smolen J.S., Landewe R., Bijlsma J., et al: Eular recommendations for the management of rheumatoid arthritis with synthetic and biological disease-modifying antirheumatic drugs: 2016 update. Ann Rheum Dis 2017; 76: pp. 960-977

38. Touma et al., 2011. Touma Z., Gladman D.D., Urowitz M.B., et al: Mycophenolate mofetil for induction treatment of lupus nephritis: a systemic review and metaanalysis. J Rheumatol 2011; 38: pp. 69-78

39. Vazquez et al., 2008. Vazquez S.R., Rondina M.T., and Pendleton R.C.: Azathioprine-induced warfarin resistance. Ann Pharmacother 2008; 42: pp. 1118-1123

40. Witt et al., 2016. Witt L.J., Demchuk C., Curran J.J., et al: Benefit of adjunctive tacrolimus in connective tissue disease-interstitial lung disease. Pulm Pharmacol Ther 2016; 36: pp. 46-52

41. Aaltonen et al., 2012. Aaltonen K.J., Virkki L.M., Malmivarra A., et al: Systematic review and meta-analysis of the efficacy and safety of existing TNF blocking agents in treatment of rheumatoid arthritis. PLOS ONE 2012

42. Baeten et al., 2015. Baeten D., Sieper J., Braun J., et al: Secukinumab, an interleukin-17A inhibitor, in ankylosing spondylitis. N Engl J Med 2015; 373: pp. 2534-2548

43. Bredemeir et al., 2014. Bredemeir M., de Oliveira F.K., and Rocha C.M.: Low- versus high-dose rituximab for rheumatoid arthritis: a systemic review and meta-analysis. Arthritis Care Res 2014; 66: pp. 228-235

44. Campbell et al., 2011. Campbell L., Chen C., Bhagat S.S., et al: Risk of adverse events including serious infections in rheumatoid arthritis patients treated with tocilizumab: a systematic literature review and meta-analysis of randomized controlled trials. Rheumatology 2011; 50: pp. 552-562

45. Chen and Flies, 2013. Chen L., and Flies D.B.: Molecular mechanisms of T cell co-stimulation and co-inhibition. Nat Rev Immunol 2013; 13: pp. 227-242

46. Cohen et al., 2006. Cohen S.B., Emery P., Greenwald M.W., et al: Rituximab for rheumatoid arthritis refractory to anti-tumor necrosis factor therapy: results of a multicenter, randomized, double-blind, placebo-controlled phase III trial evaluating primary efficacy and safety at twenty-four weeks. Arthritis Rheum 2006; 54: pp. 2793-2806

47. Dao and Cush, 2012. Dao K., and Cush J.J.: A vaccination primer for rheumatologists. Drug Safety Quarterly 2012

48. Deepak et al., 2013. Deepak P., Stobaugh D.J., Sherid M., et al: Neurological events with tumour necrosis factor alpha reported to the food and drug administration adverse event reporting system. Aliment Pharmacol Ther 2013; 38: pp. 388-396

49. Dorner and Kay, 2015. Dorner T., and Kay J.: Biosimilars in rheumatology: current perspectives and lessons learnt. Nat Rev Rheumatol 2015; 11: pp. 713-724

50. Engel et al., 2011. Engel P., Gomez-Puerta J.A., Ramos-Casals M., et al: Therapeutic targeting of B cells for rheumatic autoimmune diseases. Pharmacol Rev 2011; 6: pp. 127-156

51. Flint et al., 2016. Flint J., Panchal S., Hurrell A., et al: BSR and BHPR guideline on prescribing drugs in pregnancy and breastfeeding-Part I: standard and biologic disease modifying anti-rheumatic drugs and corticosteroids. Rheumatology 2016; 55: pp. 1693-1697

52. Genovese et al., 2015. Genovese M.C., Fleischmann R., Kivitz A.J., et al: Sarilumab plus methotrexate in patients with active rheumatoid arthritis and inadequate response to methotrexate: results of a phase III study. Arthritis Rheumatol 2015; 67: pp. 1424-1437

53. Goodman et al., 2017. Goodman S.M., Springer B., Guyatt G., et al: 2017 American College of Rheumatology/American Association of Hip and Knee Surgeons guideline for the perioperative management of antirheumatic medication in patients with rheumatic diseases undergoing elective total hip or total knee arthroplasty. Arthritis Rheumatol 2017; 69: pp. 1538-1551

54. Hoy, 2015. Hoy S.: Canakinumab: a review of its use in the management of systemic juvenile idiopathic arthritis. BioDrugs 2015; 29: pp. 133-142

55. Ilowite et al., 2014. Ilowite N.T., Prather K., Lokhnygina Y., et al: Randomized, double-blind, placebo-controlled trial of the efficacy and safety of rilonacept in the treatment of systemic juvenile idiopathic arthritis. Arthritis Rheumatol 2014; 66: pp. 2570-2579

56. Joensuu et al., 2015. Joensuu J.T., Huoponen S., Aaltonen K.J., et al: The cost-effectiveness of biologics for the treatment of rheumatoid arthritis: a systemic review. PLoS ONE 2015

57. Kavanaugh et al., 2015. Kavanaugh A., Puig L., Gottlieb A., et al: Maintenance of clinical efficacy and radiographic benefit through two years of ustekinumab in patients with active psoriatic arthritis: results from a randomized, placebo-controlled phase III trial. Arthritis Care Res 2015; 67: pp. 1739-1749

58. Kerbleski and Gottlieb, 2009. Kerbleski J.F., and Gottlieb A.B.: Dermatological complications and safety of anti-TNF treatments. Gut 2009; 58: pp. 1033-1039

59. Kremer et al., 2006. Kremer J.M., Genant H.K., Moreland L.W., et al: Effects of abatacept in patients with methotrexate-resistant active rheumatoid arthritis: a randomized trial. Ann Int Med 2006; 144: pp. 865-876

60. Lloyd et al., 2010. Lloyd S., Bujkiewicz S., Wailoo A.J., et al: The effectiveness of anti-TNF-α therapies when used sequentially in rheumatoid arthritis patients: a systematic review and meta-analysis. Rheumatology 2010; 49: pp. 2313-2321

61. Mariette et al., 2011. Mariette X., Matucci-Cerinic M., Pavelka K., et al: Malignancies associated with tumor necrosis factor inhibitors in registries and prospective observational studies: a systematic review and meta-analysis. Ann Rheum Dis 2011; 70: pp. 1895-1904

62. Mastroianni et al., 2011. Mastroianni C.M., Lichtner M., Del Borgo C., et al: Current trends in management of hepatitis B virus reactivation in the biologic therapy era. World J Gastroenterol 2011; 17: pp. 3881-3887

63. Mease et al., 2015. Mease P., McInnes I., Kirkham B., et al: Secukinumab inhibition of interleukin-17A in patients with psoriatic arthritis. N Engl J Med 2015; 373: pp. 1329-1339

64. Ortiz-Sanjuan et al., 2015. Ortiz-Sanjuan F., Blanco R., Riancho-Zarrabeitia L., et al: Efficacy of anakinra in refractory adult-onset Still's disease: multicenter study of 41 patients ane literature review. Medicine 2015; 94: pp. e1554

65. Paine and Ritchlin, 2016. Paine A., and Ritchlin C.T.: Targeting the interleukin-23/17 axis in axial spondyloarthritis. Current Opin Rheumatol 2016; 28: pp. 359-367

66. Patkar et al., 2008. Patkar N.M., Teng G.G., Curtis J.R., et al: Association of infections and tuberculosis with antitumor necrosis factor alpha therapy. Curr Opin Rheumatol 2008; 20: pp. 320-326

67. Ramos-Casals et al., 2008. Ramos-Casals M., Brito-Zeron P., Munoz S., et al: A systematic review of the off-label use of biological therapies in systemic autoimmune diseases. Medicine 2008; 87: pp. 345-364

68. Rubbert-Roth and Finckh, 2009. Rubbert-Roth A., and Finckh A.: Treatment options in rheumatoid arthritis failing TNF inhibitor therapy: a critical review. Arthritis Res Ther 2009; 11: pp. 51

69. Salliot et al., 2011. Salliot C., Finckh A., Katchamart W., et al: Indirect comparison of the efficacy of biologic antirheumatic agents in rheumatoid arthritis in patients with an inadequate response to conventional disease-modifying antirheumatic drugs or to an anti-tumor necrosis factor agent: a meta-analysis. Ann Rheum Dis 2011; 70: pp. 266-271

70. Schett et al., 2016. Schett G., Dayer J.-M., and Manger B.: Interleukin-1 function and role in rheumatic disease. Nature Rev Rheumatol 2016; 12: pp. 14-24

71. Schiff, 2011. Schiff M.: Abatacept treatment for rheumatoid arthritis. Rheumatology 2011; 50: pp. 437-449

72. Singh et al., 2015. Singh J.A., Cameron C., Noorbaloochi S., et al: Risk of serious infection in biological treatment of patients with rheumatoid arthritis: a systemic review and meta-analysis. Lancet 2015; 386: pp. 258-265

73. Singh et al., 2015. Singh J.A., Saag K.G., Bridges S.L., et al: 2015 American College of Rheumatology guideline for the treatment of rheumatoid arthritis. Arthritis Rheumatol 2016; 68: pp. 1-26

74. Smolen et al., 2008. Smolen J.S., Beaulieu A., Rubbert-Roth A., et al: Effect of interleukin-6 receptor inhibition with tocilizumab in patients with rheumatoid arthritis (OPTION study): a double-blind, placebo-controlled randomized trial. Lancet 2008; 371: pp. 987-997

75. Solomon et al., 2013. Solomon D.H., Rassen J.A., Kuriya B., et al: Heart failure risk among patients with rheumatoid arthritis starting a TNF antagonist. Ann Rheum Dis 2013; 72: pp. 1813-1818

76. Stone et al., 2010. Stone J.H., Merkel P.A., Spiera R., et al: Rituximab versus cyclophosphamide for ANCA-associated vasculitis. N Engl J Med 2010; 363: pp. 221-232

77. Stone et al., 2017. Stone J.H., Tuckwell K., Dimonaco S., et al: Trial of tocilizumab in giant cell arteritis. N Engl J Med 2017; 377: pp. 317-328

78. Tanaka and Kishimoto, 2014. Tanaka T., and Kishimoto T.: The biology and medical implications of interleukin-6. Cancer Immunol Res 2014; 2: pp. 288

79. Tarp et al., 2016. Tarp S., Amarilyo G., Foeldvari I., et al: Efficacy and safety of biological agents for systemic juvenile idiopathic arthritis: a systemic review and meta-analysis of randomized trials. Rheumatology 2016; 55: pp. 669-679

80. Tesfa et al., 2011. Tesfa D., Ajeganova S., Hagglund H., et al: Late-onset neutropenia following rituximab therapy in rheumatic diseases: association with B lymphocyte depletion and infections. Arthritis Rheumatol 2011; 63: pp. 2209-2214

81. Winthrop et al., 2009. Winthrop K.L., Chang E., Yamashita S., et al: Nontuberculosis mycobacteria infections and anti-tumor necrosis factor-α therapy. Emerg Infect Dis 2009; 15: pp. 1556-1561

82. Winthrop et al., 2013. Winthrop K.L., et al: Mycobacterial diseases and antitumor necrosis factor therapy in USA. Ann Rheum Dis 2013; 72: pp. 37-42

83. Choi et al., 2018 5. Choi H., Neogi T., Stamp L., Dalbeth N., and Terkeltaub R.: Implications of the cardiovascular safety of febuxostat and allopurinol in patients with gout and cardiovascular morbidities (CARES) trial and associated FDA public safety alert. Arthritis Rheumatol 2018.

84. Colchicine. In Micromedex (Columbia Basin College Library ed.) [Electronic version]. Greenwood Village, CO: Truven Health Analytics.

85. Khanna et al., 2012. Khanna D., et al: American College of Rheumatology Guidelines for Management of gout. Part 1. Systematic nonpharmacologic and pharmacologic therapeutic approaches to hyperuricemia. Arth Care Res 2012; 64: pp. 1431-1446

86. Khanna et al., 2012. Khanna D., Khanna P.P., Fitzgerald J.D., et al: American College of Rheumatology guidelines for management of gout. Part 2: therapy and antiinflammatory prophylaxis of acute gouty arthritis. Arthritis Care Res 2012; 64: pp. 1447-1461

87. Pegloticase injection label.

88. Slobodnick et al., 2015. Slobodnick A., Shah B., Pillinger M.H., and Krasnokutsky S.: Colchicine: old and new. Am J Med 2015; 128: pp. 461-470

89. Stamp et al., 2014. Stamp L.K., Merriman T.R., Barclay M.L., Singh J.A., Roberts R.L., Wright D.F., and Dalbeth N.: Impaired response or insufficient dosage? Examining the potential causes of "inadequate response" to allopurinol in the treatment of gout. Semin Arthritis Rheum 2014; 44: pp. 170-174

90. Stamp et al., 2011. Stamp L.K., O'Donnell J.L., Zhang M., et al: Using allopurinol above the dose based on creatinine clearance is effective and safe in patients with chronic gout, including those with renal impairment. Arthritis Rheum 2011; 63: pp. 412-421

91. Stamp et al., 2012. Stamp L.K., Taylor W.J., Jones P.B., et al: Starting dose is a risk factor for allopurinol hypersensitivity syndrome: a proposed safe starting dose of allopurinol. Arthritis Rheum 2012; 64: pp. 2529-2536

92. Terkeltaub et al., 2010. Terkeltaub R.A., Furst D.E., Bennett K., et al: High versus low dosing of oral colchicine for early acute gout flare. Arthritis Rheum 2010; 62: pp. 1060-1068

93. Terkeltaub et al., 2011. Terkeltaub R.A., Furst D.E., Digiacinto J.L., et al: Novel evidence-based colchicine dose-reduction algorithm to predict and prevent colchicine toxicity in the presence of cytochrome P450 3A4/P-glycoprotein inhibitors. Arthritis Rheum 2011; 63: pp. 2226-2237

94. Adler et al., 2016. Adler R.A., Fuleihan G.E.-H., Bauer D.C., et al: Managing osteoporosis in patients on long-term bisphosphonate treatment: report of a task force of the American Society for Bone and Mineral Research. J Bone Min Res 2016; 31: pp. 16-35

95. Adler, 2018. Adler R.A.: Management of endocrine disease: atypical femoral fractures: risks and benefits of long-term treatment of osteoporosis with anti-resorptive therapy. Eur J Endocrinol 2018; 178: pp. R81-R87

96. Anastasilakis et al., 2017. Anastasilakis A.D., Polyzos S.A., Makras P., et al: Clinical features of 24 patients with rebound-associated vertebral fractures after denosumab discontinuation: systematic review and additional cases. J Bone Min Res 2017; 32: pp. 1291-1296

97. Axelsson et al., 2017. Axelsson K.F., Nilsson A.G., Wedel H., et al: Association between alendronate use and hip fracture risk in older patients using oral prednisolone. JAMA 2017; 318: pp. 146-155

98. Bindon et al., 2018. Bindon B., Adams W., Balasubramanian N., et al: Osteoporosis fractures during bisphosphonate drug holidays. Endocrine Pract 2018; 24: pp. 163-169

99. Black and Rosen, 2016. Black D.M., and Rosen C.J.: Postmenopausal osteoporosis. N Engl J Med 2016; 374: pp. 254-262

100. Bone et al., 2017. Bone H.G., Wagman R.B., Brandi M.L., et al: 10 years of denosumab treatment in postmenopausal women with osteoporosis: results from the phase 3 randomized FREEDOM trial and open label extension. Lancet Diabet Endocrinol 2017; 5: pp. 513-523

101. Bonnick et al., 2001. Bonnick S., Johnston C.C., Kleerekoper M., et al: Importance of precision in bone density measurements. J Clin Densitometry 2001; 4: pp. 1-6

102. Buckley et al., 2017. Buckley L., Guyatt G., Fink H.A., et al: 2017 American College of Rheumatology guideline for the prevention and treatment of glucocorticoid-induced osteoporosis. Arthritis Rheum 2017; 69: pp. 1521-1537

103. Camacho et al., 2016. Camacho P.M., Petak S.M., Binkley N., et al: American Association of Clinical Endocrinologists and American College of Endocrinology clinical practice guidelines for the diagnosis and treatment of postmenopausal osteoporosis – 2016. Endocrine Pract 2016; 22: pp. 1-42

104. Chapurlat, 2017. Chapurlat R.: Effects and management of denosumab discontinuation. Joint Bone Spine 2017

105. Chung et al., 2016. Chung M., Tang A.M., Fu Z., Wang D.D., and Newberry S.J.: Calcium intake and cardiovascular disease risk: an updated systematic review and meta-analysis. Ann Intern Med 2016; 165: pp. 856-866

106. Cosman et al., 2016. Cosman F., Crittenden D.B., Adachi J.D., et al: Romosozumab treatment in postmenopausal women with osteoporosis. (EVENITY). N Engl J Med 2016; 375: pp. 1532-1543

107. Cosman et al., 2017. Cosman F., Miller P.D., Williams C.G., et al: Eighteen months of treatment with subcutaneous abaloparatide followed by 6 months of treatment with alendronate in postmenopausal women with osteoporosis: results of the ACTIVExtend trial. Mayo Clin Proc 2017; 92: pp. 200-210

108. Cosman et al., 2017. Cosman F., Nieves J.W., and Dempster D.W.: Treatment sequence matters: anabolic and antiresorptive therapy for osteoporosis. J Bone Min Res 2017; 32: pp. 198-202

109. Crandall et al., 2014. Crandall C.J., Newberry S.J., Diamant A., et al: Comparative effectiveness of pharmacologic treatments to prevent fractures: an updated systematic review. Ann Intern Med 2014; 161: pp. 711-723

110. Cummings et al., 2017. Cummings S.R., Cosman F., Lewiecki E.M., et al: Goal-directed treatment for osteoporosis: a progress report from the ASBMR-NOF working group on goal-directed treatment for osteoporosis. J Bone Min Res 2017; 32: pp. 3-10

111. Cummings et al., 2018. Cummings S.R., Ferrari S., Eastell R., et al: Vertebral fractures after discontinuation of denosumab: a post hoc analysis of the randomized placebo-controlled FREEDOM trial and its extension. J Bone Min Res 2018; 33: pp. 190-197

112. Dawson-Hughes and Bischoff-Ferrari, 2007. Dawson-Hughes B., and Bischoff-Ferrari H.A.: Therapy of osteoporosis with calcium and vitamin D. J Bone Min Res 2007; 22: pp. V59-63

113. Eastell and Szulc, 2017. Eastell R., and Szulc P.: Use of bone turnover markers in postmenopausal osteoporosis. Osteoporosis treatment: recent developments and ongoing challenges. Lancet Diabetes Endocrinol 2017; 5: pp. 908-923

114. Holick, 2007. Holick M.F.: Vitamin D deficiency. N Engl J Med 2007; 357: pp. 266-281

115. Kendler et al., 2017 9. Kendler D.L., Marin F., Zerbini C.A.F., et al: Effects of teriparatide and risedronate on new fractures in post-menopausal women with severe osteoporosis (VERO): a multicentre, double-blind, double-dummy, randomised controlled trial. Lancet 2017

116. Khan et al., 2015. Khan A.A., Morrison A., Hanley D.A., et al: Diagnosis and management of osteonecrosis of the jaw: a systematic review and international consensus. J Bone Min Res 2015; 30: pp. 3-23

117. Kosla and Hofbauer, 2017. Kosla S., and Hofbauer L.: Osteoporosis treatment: recent developments and ongoing challenges. Lancet Diabetes Endocrinol 2017; 5: pp. 898-907

118. Langdahl et al., 2017. Langdahl B.L., Libanati C., Crittenden D.B., et al: Romosozumab (sclerostin monoclonal antibody) versus teriparatide in postmenopausal women with osteoporosis transitioning from oral bisphosphonate therapy: a randomised, open-label, phase 3 trial. Lancet 2017; 390: pp. 1585-1594

119. Leder et al., 2015. Leder B.Z., O'Dee L.S., Zanchetta J.R., et al: Effects of abaloparatide, a human parathyroid hormone-related peptide analog, on bone mineral density in postmenopausal women with osteoporosis. J Clin Endocrinol Metab 2015

120. Leder et al., 2014. Leder B.Z., Tsai J.N., Uihlein A.V., et al: Two years of denosumab and teriparatide administration in postmenopausal women with osteoporosis (the DATA Extension Study): a randomized controlled trial. J Clin Endocrinol Metab 2014; 99: pp. 1694-1700

121. Leder et al., 2015. Leder B.Z., Tsai J.N., Uihlein A.V., et al: Denosumab and teriparatide transitions in postmenopausal osteoporosis (the DATA-Switch study): extension of a randomized controlled trial. Lancet 2015; 336: pp. 1147-1155

122. Lewiecki, 2003. Lewiecki E.M.: Nonresponders to osteoporosis therapy. J Clin Densitometry 2003; 6: pp. 307-314

123. Lewiecki et al., 2013. Lewiecki M., Cummings S.R., and Cosman F.: Treat-to-target for osteoporosis: is now the time? J Clin Endocrinol Metab 2013; 98: pp. 946-953

124. Lewis et al., 2015. Lewis J.R., Radavelli-Bagatini S., Rejnmark L., et al: The effects of calcium supplementation on verified coronary heart disease hospitalization and death in postmenopausal women: a collaborative meta-analysis of randomized controlled trials. J Bone Min Res 2015; 30: pp. 165-175

125. Lloyd et al., 2017. Lloyd A.A., Gludovatz B., Riedel C., et al: Atypical fracture with long-term bisphosphonate therapy is associated with altered cortical composition and reduced fracture resistance. Proc Natl Acad Sci USA 2017; 114: pp. 8722-8727

126. Long, 2011. Long F.: Building stronger bones: molecular regulation of the osteoblast lineage. Nat Rev Mol Cell Biol 2011; 13: pp. 27-38

127. Malouf-Sierra et al., 2017. Malouf-Sierra J., Tarantino U., García-Hernández P.A., et al: Effect of teriparatide or risedronate in elderly patients with a recent pertrochanteric hip fracture: final results of a 78-week randomized clinical trial. J Bone Miner Res 2017; 32: pp. 1040-1051

128. Marie and Cohen-Solal, 2018. Marie P.J., and Cohen-Solal M.: The expanding life and functions of osteogenic cells: from simple bone-making cells to multifunctional cells and beyond. J Bone Min Res 2018; 33: pp. 199-210

129. McClung et al., 2013. McClung M.R., Lewiecki E.M., Geller M.L., et al: Effect of denosumab on bone mineral density and biochemical markers of bone turnover: 8 year results of a phase 2 clinical trial. Osteoporosis Int 2013; 24: pp. 227-235

130. McClung, 2016. McClung M.R.: Cancel the denosumab holiday. Osteoporosis Int 2016; 27: pp. 1677-1682

131. McClung et al., 2017. McClung M.R., Wagman R.B., Miller P.D., Wang A., and Lewiecki E.M.: Observations following discontinuation of long-term denosumab therapy. Osteoporosis Int 2017; 28: pp. 1723-1732

132. McClung, 2017. McClung M.R.: Clinical utility of anti-sclerostin antibodies. Bone 2017; 96: pp. 3-7

133. McClung, 2017. McClung M.R.: Using osteoporosis therapies in combination. Curr Osteoporosis Rep 2017; 15: pp. 343-352

134. Miller et al., 2016. Miller P.D., Pannacciulli N., Brown J.P., et al: Denosumab or zoledronic acid in postmenopausal women with osteoporosis previously treated with oral bisphosphonates. J Clin Endocrinol Metab 2016; 101: pp. 3163-3170

135. Miller et al., 2016. Miller P.D., Hattersley G., Riis B.J., et al: Effect of abaloparatide vs placebo on new vertebral fractures in postmenopausal women with osteoporosis: a randomized clinical trial. ACTIVE trial) JAMA 2016; 316: pp. 722-733

136. Olivier et al., 2017. Olivier L., Gonzalez-Rodriguez E., Stoli D., Hans D., and Aubry-Rozier B.: Severe rebound-associated vertebral fractures after denosumab discontinuation: 9 clinical cases report. J Clin Endocrinol Metab 2017; 102: pp. 354-358

137. Park-Wyllie et al., 2011. Park-Wyllie L., Mamdani M.M., Juurink D.N., et al: Bisphosphonate use and the risk of subtrochanteric or femoral shaft fractures in older women. JAMA 2011; 305: pp. 783-789

138. Qaseem et al., 2017. Qaseem A., Forciea M.A., McLean R.M., and Denberg T.D.: Treatment of low bone density or osteoporosis to prevent fractures in men and women: a clinical practice guideline update from the American College of Physicians. Ann Intern Med 2017; 166: pp. 818-839

139. Rothman et al., 2017. Rothman M.S., Lewiecki E.M., and Miller P.D.: Bone density testing is the best way to monitor osteoporosis. Am J Med 2017; 130: pp. 1133-1134

140. Ruggiero et al., 2014. Ruggiero S.L., Dodson T.B., Fantasia L., et al: American Association of Oral and Maxillofacial Surgeons position paper on medication-related osteonecrosis of the jaw – 2014 update. J Oral Maxillofac Surg 2014; 72: pp. 1938-1956

141. Saag et al., 2017. Saag K.G., Petersen J., and Brandi M.L.: Romosozumab or alendronate for fracture prevention in women with osteoporosis. (EVENITY). N Engl J Med 2017; 377: pp. 1417-1427

142. Saag et al., 2018. Saag K.G., Wagman R.B., Geusens P., et al: Denosumab versus risedronate in glucocorticoid-induced osteoporosis: a multicentre, randomized, double-blind, active-controlled, double-dummy, non-inferiority study. Lancet Diabetes Endocrinol 2018; 6: pp. 445-454

143. Shane et al., 2014. Shane E., Burr D., Abrahamsen B., et al: Atypical subtrochanteric and diaphyseal femoral fractures: second report of a task force of the American Society for Bone and Mineral Research. J Bone Min Res 2014; 29: pp. 1-23

144. Buttgereit et al., 2013. Buttgereit F., Mehta D., Kirwan J., et al: Low-dose prednisone chronotherapy for rheumatoid arthritis: a randomized clinical trial (CAPRA-2). Ann Rheum Dis 2013; 72: pp. 204-210

145. Curtis et al., 2006. Curtis J.R., Westfall A.O., Allison J., et al: Population-based assessment of adverse events associated with long-term glucocorticoid use. Arthritis Rheum 2006; 55: pp. 420-426

146. Hench et al., 1949. Hench P.S., Kendall E.C., Slocumb C.H., et al: The effect of a hormone of the adrenal cortex (17 hydroxy-11-dehydrocorticosterone: compound E) and of pituitary adrenocorticotropic hormone on rheumatoid arthritis: preliminary report. Proc Staff Meet Mayo Clin 1949; 24: pp. 181-197

147. Richter et al., 2002. Richter B., Neises G., and Clar C.: Glucocorticoid withdrawal schemes in chronic medical disorders. A systemic review. Endocrinol Metab Clin North Am 2002; 31: pp. 751-778

148. Saag and Buttgereit, 2019. Saag K., and Buttgereit F.: Systemic glucocorticoid therapy in rheumatology. In Hochberg M.C. (eds): Rheumatology, 7th ed. Philadelphia: Elsevier, 2019. pp. 488-498

149. Stahn and Buttgereit, 2008. Stahn C., and Buttgereit F.: Genomic and nongenomic effects of glucocorticoids. Nat Clin Pract Rheumatol 2008; 4: pp. 525-533

150. Strehl et al., 2016. Strehl C., Bijlsma J.W., de Wit M., et al: Defining conditions where long-term glucocorticoid treatment has an acceptably low level of harm to facilitate implementation of existing recommendations: viewpoints from an EULAR task force. Ann Rheum Dis 2016; 75: pp. 952-957

151. Waljee et al., 2017. Waljee A.K., Rogers M.A., Lin P., et al: Short term use of oral corticosteroids and related harms among adults in the United States: population based cohort study. BMJ 2017; 357: pp. 1415

152. Winthrop and Baddley, 2018. Winthrop K.L., and Baddley J.W.: Pneumocystis and glucocorticoid use: to prophylax or not to prophylax (and when?); that is the question. Ann Rheum Dis 2018; 77: pp. 631-633

153. Bally and Dendukuri, 2017 9. Bally M., and Dendukuri N.: Risk of acute myocardial infarction with NSAIDs in real world use: bayesian meta-analysis of individual patient data. BMJ 2017; 357: pp. 1909

154. Bhala N (on behalf of NSAID Trialists Collaboration), 2013. Vascular and upper gastrointestinal effects of non-steroidal anti-inflammatory drugs: meta-analyses of individual participant data from randomized trials. Lancet 2013; 382: pp. 769-779

155. Capone et al., 2005. Capone M.L., Sciulli M.G., Tacconelli S., et al: Pharmacodynamic interaction of naproxen with low-dose aspirin in healthy subjects. J. Am. Coll. Cardiol. 2005; 45: pp. 1295-1301

156. Castelli and Petrone, 2017. Castelli G., and Petrone A.: Rates of nonsteroidal anti-inflammatory drug use in patients with established cardiovascular disease: a retrospective, cross-sectional study from NHANES 2009-2010. Am J Cardiovasc Drugs 2017 Jun; 17: pp. 243-249

157. Catella-Lawson et al., 2001. Catella-Lawson F., Reilly M.P., Kapoor S.C., et al: Cyclooxygenase inhibitors and the antiplatelet effects of aspirin. N Engl J Med 2001; 345: pp. 1809-1817

158. Chan et al., 2001. Chan F.K., Chung S.C., Suen B.Y., et al: Preventing recurrent upper gastrointestinal bleeding in patients with Helicobacter pylori infection who are taking low-dose aspirin or naproxen. N Engl J Med 2001; 344: pp. 967-973

159. Chan et al., 2004. Chan F.K., Hung L.C., Suen B.Y., et al: Celecoxib versus diclofenac plus omeprazole in high risk patients: results of a randomized double-blind trial. Gastroenterology 2004; 127: pp. 1038-1043

160. Chan et al., 2007. Chan F.K., Wong V.W., Suen B.Y., et al: Combination of a COX-2 inhibitor and a proton pump inhibitor for the prevention of recurrent ulcer bleeding in patients at very high risk: a double blind, randomized trial. Lancet 2007; 369: pp. 1621-1626

161. Davis and Lee, 2017. Davis J.S., and Lee H.Y.: Use of non-steroidal anti-inflammatory drugs in US adults: changes over time and by demographic. Open Heart 2017

162. Garcia Rodriquez et al., 2008. Garcia Rodriquez L.A., Tacconelli S., and Patrignani P.: Role of dose potency in the prediction of risk of myocardial infarction associated with nonsteroidal anti-inflammatory drugs in the general population. J Am Coll Cardiol 2008; 52: pp. 1628-1636

163. Lanas, 2005. Lanas A.: Gastrointestinal injury from NSAID therapy: how to reduce the risk of complications. Postgrad Med 2005; 117: pp. 13

164. Lanza et al., 2009. Lanza F.L., Chan F.K., and Quigley E.M.: Guidelines for prevention of NSAID-related ulcer complications. Am J Gastroenter 2009; 104: pp. 728-738

165. McAdam et al., 1999. McAdam B.F., Catella-Lawson F., Mardini I.A., et al: Systemic biosynthesis of prostacyclin by COX-2: the human pharmacology of a selective inhibitor of COX-2. Proc Natl Acad Sci USA 1999; 96: pp. 272-277

166. Nissen and Yeomans, 2016. Nissen S.E., and Yeomans N.D.: Cardiovascular safety of celecoxib, naproxen, or ibuprofen for arthritis. N Engl J Med 2016; 375: pp. 2519-2529

167. Schjerning et al., 2011. Schjerning O.A.M., Fosbel E.L., Lindhardsen J., et al: Duration of treatment with NSAIDs and impact on risk of death and recurrent myocardial infarction in patients with prior myocardial infarction: a nationwide cohort study. Circulation 2011; 123: pp. 2226-2235

168. Zhou and Freedman, 2014. Zhou Y., and Freedman A.N.: Trends in the use of aspirin and nonsteroidal anti-inflammatory drugs in the general U.S. population. Pharmacoepidemiol Drug Saf 2014 Jan; 23: pp. 43-50

169. Andreoli et al., 2017. Andreoli L., Bertsias G.K., Agmon-Levin N., et al: EULAR recommendations for women's health and the management of family planning, assisted reproduction, pregnancy and menopause in patients with systemic lupus erythematosus and/or antiphospholipid syndrome. Ann Rheum Dis 2017; 76: pp. 476-485

170. Buyon et al., 2015. Buyon J.P., Kim M.Y., Guerra M.M., et al: Predictors of pregnancy outcomes in patients with lupus: a cohort study. Ann Int Med 2015; 163: pp. 153-163

171. Empson et al., 2002. Empson M., Lassere M., Craig J.C., and Scott J.R.: Recurrent pregnancy loss with antiphospholipid antibody: a systematic review of therapeutic trials. Obstet 2002; 99: pp. 135-144

172. Garcia and Erkan, 2018. Garcia D., and Erkan D.: Diagnosis and management of the antiphospholipid syndrome. N Engl J Med 2018; 378: pp. 2010-2021

173. Izmirly et al., 2012. Izmirly P.A., Costedoat-Chalumeau N., Pisoni C.N., et al: Maternal use of hydroxychloroquine is associated with a reduced risk of recurrent SSA associated cardiac manifestations of neonatal lupus syndrome. Circulation 2012; 126: pp. 76-82

174. Jakobsson et al., 2016. Jakobsson G.L., Stephansson O., Askling J., and Jacobsson L.T.H.: Pregnancy outcomes in patients with ankylosing spondylitis: a nationwide register study. Ann Rheum Dis 2016; 75: pp. 1838-1842

175. Lightstone and Hladunewich, 2017. Lightstone L., and Hladunewich M.A.: Lupus nephritis and pregnancy: concerns and management. Semin Nephrol 2017; 37: pp. 347-353

176. Machen and Clowse, 2017. Machen L., and Clowse M.E.: Vasculitis and pregnancy. Rheum Dis Clin North Am 2017; 43: pp. 239-247

177. Marder et al., 2016. Marder W., Littlejohn E.A., and Somers E.C.: Pregnancy and autoimmune connective tissue diseases. Best Pract Res Clin Rheumatol 2016; 30: pp. 63-80

178. Miyakis et al., 2006. Miyakis S., Lockshin M.D., Atsumi T., et al: International consensus statement on an update of the classification criteria for definite antiphospholipid syndrome (APS). J Thomb Haemost 2006; 4: pp. 295-306

179. Noviani et al., 2016. Noviani M., Wasserman S., and Clowse M.E.: Breastfeeding in mothers with systemic lupus erythematosus. Lupus 2016; 41: pp. 476-481

180. Nukumizu et al., 2012. Nukumizu L.A., et al: Gonadal function in male patients with ankylosing spondylitis. Scand J Rheumatol 2012; 41: pp. 476-481

181. Østensen et al., 2012. Østensen M., Villiger P.M., and Förger F.: Interaction of pregnancy and autoimmune rheumatic disease. Autoimmun Rev 2012; 11: pp. A437-A446

182. Polachek et al., 2017. Polachek A., Li S., Polachek I.S., Chandran V., and Gladman D.: Psoriatic arthritis disease activity during pregnancy and the first-year postpartum. Semin Arthritis Rheum 2017; 46: pp. 740-745

183. Sammaritano, 2017. Sammaritano L.R.: Contraception in patients with rheumatic disease. Rheum Dis Clin North Am 2017; 43: pp. 173-188

184. Uzunasian et al., 2014. Uzunasian D., et al: No appreciable decrease in fertility in Behçet's syndrome. Rheumatology (Oxford) 2014; 53: pp. 828-833

185. van den Brandt et al., 2017. van den Brandt S., Zbinden A., Baeten D., Villiger P.M., Østensen M., and Forger F.: Risk factors for flare and treatment of disease flares during pregnancy in rheumatoid arthritis and axial spondyloarthritis patients. Arthritis Res Ther 2017; 19: pp. 64

186. Young and Khanna, 2015. Young A., and Khanna D.: Systemic sclerosis: commonly asked questions by rheumatologists. J Clin Rheumatol 2015; 21: pp. 149-155

187. Khanna et al, 2021. Reducing Immunogenicity of Pegloticase with Concomitant Use of Mycophenolate Mofetil in Patients with Refractory Gout: A Phase II, Randomized, Double-Blind, Placebo-Controlled Trial. Arthritis & Rheumatology, August 2021; 73(8): 1523-1532.

188. Furie et al, 2020. Two-Year, Randomized, Controlled Trial of Belimumab in Lupus Nephritis. New England Journal of Medicine, September 2020; 383: 1117-1128.

189. Werth et al, 2018. A phase 2 study of safety and efficacy of lenabasum (JBT-101), a cannabinoid receptor type 2 agonist, in refractory skin-predominant dermatomyositis. Annals of the Rheumatic Diseases 2018; 77:763-764.

190. Kalunian et al. A Phase II study of the efficacy and safety of rontalizumab (rhuMAb interferon-alpha) in patients with systemic lupus erythematosus (ROSE). Annals of Rheumatic Disease, January 2016; 75(1): 196-202.

191. Khamashta et al. Sifalimumab, an anti-interferon-alpha monoclonal antibody, in moderate to severe systemic lupus erythematosus: a randomized, double-blind, placebo-controlled study. Annals of the Rheumatic Diseases, 2016; 75: 1909-1916.

192. Furie et al. Anifrolumab, an Anti-Interferon-alpha Receptor Monoclonal Antibody, in Moderate-to-Severe Systemic Lupus Erythematosus. Arthritis & Rheumatology, 2017; 69(2): 376-386.

193. Smolen et al. Olokizumab versus Placebo or Adalimumab in Rheumatoid Arthritis. NEJM 387;8, August 2022.

194. Levine, Todd. Treating refractory dermatomyositis or polymyositis with adrenocorticotropic hormone gel: a retrospective case series. Drug Design, Development and Therapy, 2012: 6(133-139).

195. Patel et al. Melanocortin receptors as novel effectors of macrophage responses in inflammation. Frontiers in Immunology. September 2011, Volume 2, Article 41.

196. Mease PJ, Deodhar AA, van der Heijde D, Behrens F, Kivitz AJ, Neal J, Kim J, Singhal S, Nowak M, Banerjee S. Efficacy and safety of selective TYK2 inhibitor, deucravacitinib, in a phase II trial in psoriatic arthritis. Ann Rheum Dis. 2022 Jun;81(6):815-822.

197. Nogueira M, Puig L, Torres T. JAK Inhibitors for Treatment of Psoriasis: Focus on Selective TYK2 Inhibitors. Drugs. 2020 Mar;80(4):341-352.

198. Gonciarz M, Pawlak-Buś K, Leszczyński P, Owczarek W. TYK2 as a therapeutic target in the treatment of autoimmune and inflammatory diseases. Immunotherapy. 2021 Sep;13(13):1135-1150.

199. Wrobleski ST, Moslin R, Lin S, Zhang Y, Spergel S, Kempson J, Tokarski JS, Strnad J, Zupa-Fernandez A, Cheng L, Shuster D, Gillooly K, Yang X, Heimrich E, McIntyre KW, Chaudhry C, Khan J, Ruzanov M, Tredup J, Mulligan D, Xie D, Sun H, Huang C, D'Arienzo C, Aranibar N, Chiney M, Chimalakonda A, Pitts WJ, Lombardo L, Carter PH, Burke JR, Weinstein DS. Highly Selective Inhibition of Tyrosine Kinase 2 (TYK2) for the Treatment of Autoimmune Diseases: Discovery of the Allosteric Inhibitor BMS-986165. J Med Chem. 2019 Oct 24;62(20):8973-8995.

200. Akram MS, Pery N, Butler L, Shafiq MI, Batool N, Rehman MFU, Grahame-Dunn LG, Yetisen AK. Challenges for biosimilars: focus on rheumatoid arthritis. Crit Rev Biotechnol. 2021 Feb;41(1):121-153. doi: 10.1080/07388551.2020.1830746. Epub 2020 Oct 11. PMID: 33040628.

201. Janjigian YY, Bissig M, Curigliano G, Coppola J, Latymer M. Talking to patients about biosimilars. Future Oncol. 2018 Oct;14(23):2403-2414. doi: 10.2217/fon-2018-0044. Epub 2018 Jun 1. PMID: 29856243.

202. Agboton C, Salameh J. Biosimilars in chronic inflammatory diseases: facts and remaining questions 5 years after their introduction in Europe. Expert Opin Biol Ther. 2022 Feb;22(2):157-167. doi: 10.1080/14712598.2021.1963435. Epub 2021 Aug 9. PMID: 34338115.

203. Kay J. Overcoming barriers to biosimilars in inflammatory arthritis. Nat Rev Rheumatol. 2020 Feb;16(2):65-66. doi: 10.1038/s41584-019-0359-7. PMID: 31873190.

204. Smolen JS, Goncalves J, Quinn M, Benedetti F, Lee JY. Era of biosimilars in rheumatology: reshaping the healthcare environment. RMD Open. 2019 May 21;5(1):e000900. doi: 10.1136/rmdopen-2019-000900. PMID: 31245050; PMCID: PMC6560670.

205. Hetland ML. Rheumatology: biosimilars are here to stay. Rheumatology (Oxford). 2022 Apr 11;61(4):1312-1313. doi: 10.1093/rheumatology/keab663. PMID: 34559204.

206. Dey M, Zhao SS, Moots RJ. Anti-TNF biosimilars in rheumatology: the end of an era? Expert Opin Biol Ther. 2021 Jan;21(1):29-36. doi: 10.1080/14712598.2020.1802421. Epub 2020 Aug 12. PMID: 32735158.

207. Edwards CJ, Bellinvia S. Biosimilars. Lupus. 2020 May;29(6):525-532. doi: 10.1177/0961203320910797. Epub 2020 Mar 18. PMID: 32188301.

208. McInnes IB, Asahina A, Coates LC, Landewé R, Merola JF, Ritchlin CT, Tanaka Y, Gossec L, Gottlieb AB, Warren RB, Ink B, Assudani D, Bajracharya R, Shende V, Coarse J, Mease PJ. Bimekizumab in patients with psoriatic arthritis, naive to biologic treatment: a randomised, double-blind, placebo-controlled, phase 3 trial (BE OPTIMAL). Lancet. 2023 Jan 7;401(10370):25-37.

209. Noaiseh G, Sivils KL, Campbell K, Idokogi J, Lo KH, Liva SG, Leu JH, Dhatt H, Ma K, Leonardo S, Li H, Hubbard JJ, Gottenberg JE. Efficacy and safety of nipocalimab in patients with moderate-to-severe Sjögren's disease (DAHLIAS): a randomised, phase 2, placebo-controlled, double-blind trial. Lancet. 2025 Nov 22;406(10518):2435-2448.

210. Dörner T, Bowman SJ, Fox R, Mariette X, Papas A, Grader-Beck T, Fisher BA, Barcelos F, De Vita S, Schulze-Koops H, Moots RJ, Junge G, Woznicki J, Sopala M, Avrameas A, Luo WL, Hueber W. Safety and Efficacy of Ianalumab in Patients With Sjögren's Disease: 52-Week Results From a Randomized, Placebo-Controlled, Phase 2b Dose-Ranging Study. Arthritis Rheumatol. 2025 May;77(5):560-570.

211. Vleugels RA, Paik JJ, Bauer Ventura I, Mangold AR, Gandiga PC, Haemel A, Chinoy H, Hussain YM, Sivakumar K, Zoltan G, Lee EB, Bozan F, Hsu CY, Femia A, Dimachkie MM, Min MS, Mozaffar T, Charles-Schoeman C, Fernandez DR, Onajin O, Marques R, Marder G, Ernste F, Schiopu E, Sluzevich J, Pearson D, Lindsey S, Luggen M, Bubb MR, Boh E, Maganti R, Heinlen L, Shaw KS, Cascino MD, Mudd PN Jr, Vencovsky J, Fernandez AP, Fiorentino D, Christopher-Stine L, Werth VP, Aggarwal R; VALOR Investigators. A Phase 3 Trial of Brepocitinib in Dermatomyositis. N Engl J Med. 2026 Mar 28. doi: 10.105

212. Schett G, Mackensen A, Mougiakakos D. CAR T-cell therapy in autoimmune diseases. Lancet. 2023 Nov 25;402(10416):2034-2044. doi: 10.1016/S0140-6736(23)01126-1. Epub 2023 Sep 22. PMID: 37748491.

213. Mackensen A, Müller F, Mougiakakos D, Böltz S, Wilhelm A, Aigner M, Völkl S, Simon D, Kleyer A, Munoz L, Kretschmann S, Kharboutli S, Gary R, Reimann H, Rösler W, Uderhardt S, Bang H, Herrmann M, Ekici AB, Buettner C, Habenicht KM, Winkler TH, Krönke G, Schett G. Anti-CD19 CAR T cell therapy for refractory systemic lupus erythematosus. Nat Med. 2022 Oct;28(10):2124-2132.

214. Medscape. https://www.medscape.com

About the Author

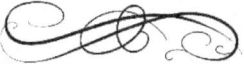

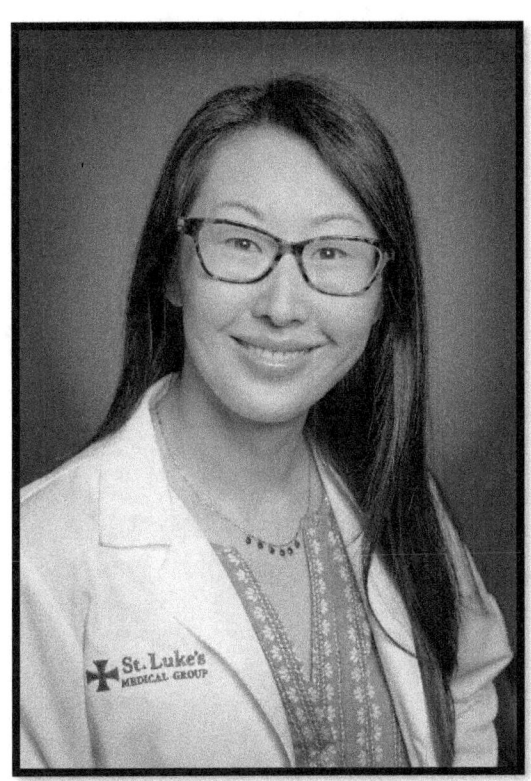

Donica Liu Baker, MD, FACR is a rheumatologist practicing the art of medicine in her beloved hometown of St. Louis, Missouri. As a Kinesiology major in college at the University of Michigan-Ann Arbor, she developed an early passion for helping patients improve their mobility, which evolved into an interest in arthritis and autoimmune diseases.

She completed most of her medical education, including rheumatology fellowship, at the University of Missouri in Columbia. For her, the best part of being in medicine is having a window of perspective to understand humanity from all walks of life, and getting to see points of view that are different from her own.

Creative writing is one of her passions and she is a blog writer for arthritis websites. She enjoys spending time with her family, yoga, piano, hiking with her dogs Sasha and Coco, and exploring activities around St. Louis city.

www.ingramcontent.com/pod-product-compliance
Lightning Source LLC
Chambersburg PA
CBHW081433220526
45466CB00008B/2371